Preface

Air travel has demolished the barriers of distance and has eased the passage of infection from distant lands. The physician of today can no longer ignore the problems of infection but few undergraduates have the opportunity to study infectious diseases by the bedside and many postgraduates are unfamiliar with infections still widely prevalent in many parts of the world. Moreover, the increasing numbers of immune-deficient patients have encouraged the spread of opportunistic micro-organisms and added a new dimension to the age-old problems of infection.

This Atlas is designed to test the student's knowledge of commonplace infections, which form such an important part of everyday practice, and provide a challenge to the more experienced physician who is likely to encounter unusual and exotic infections in travellers. Emphasis has been placed upon the clinical aspects of infection but the understanding of disease would be incomplete without some knowledge of the basic microbiology and pathology, so we have included relevant questions on these subjects. An index has been provided to enable the reader to use the tests in a constructive manner by relating the individual photographs and text on a single disease.

Acknowledgements

It would have been impossible to cover such a wide range of infections without the generous support of many friends and colleagues who have provided illustrations from their collections and we are most grateful to: the late Dr E.H. Brown 37, 169; Mr D. Downton 186; Dr T.H. Flewett 43; Dr W.M. Jamieson 105; Mr Martin Jones 123; Dr T. Kawasaki 19, 49; Dr S.G. Lamb 41, 117; Dr J.J. Linehan 150; Dr G.D.W. McKendrick 65, 112, 187; the late Dr E.P. O'Sullivan 58, 124; Dr J.D.J. Parker 63; Dr H.G. Prentice 120; Dr J.I. Pugh 127; Dr I. Sarkany 184, 185; Professor D.I.H. Simpson 79, 168; Dr J. Stevenson 89, 143; the late Dr R.N.P. Sutton 35; Dr Frances Tatnell 31; Dr R.V. Walley 141; Dr D.A. Warrell 22, 110, 113, Dr P. Welsby 130, 196; Dr P.H.A. Willcox 199.

Some of the illustrations have been obtained from members of the former Association for the Study of Infectious Diseases to whom we are most grateful. Every effort has been made to identify the source of the illustrations but if any mistakes have been made we offer our sincere apologies.

1 A young girl developed painful blisters on her finger.
(a) What is the diagnosis?
(b) Is this a primary infection?
(c) Would there be recurrent lesions on her finger?
(d) Is this condition related to occupation in adults?

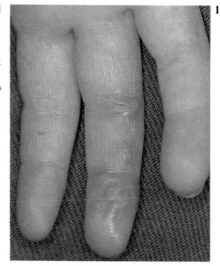

2 A worker in a duck-processing plant developed an influenzal-type illness with severe headache and myalgia, persistent dry cough and breathlessness. His spleen was palpable.
(a) What does his chest X-ray show?
(b) What is the probable diagnosis?
(c) What is the causative organism?
(d) How could the diagnosis be confirmed?
(e) What is the source of the infection?

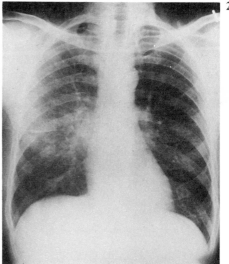

3

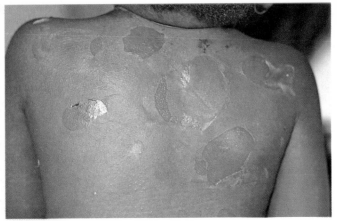

3 A young boy presented with high fever, generalised rash, conjunctivitis, stomatitis and urethritis; very painful skin with large raw areas where the necrotic epidermis had slid off the underlying layers.
(a) What is the differential diagnosis?
(b) What is the aetiology?
(c) What is the sign illustrated?
(d) What is the prognosis?

4 Three weeks after visiting Pakistan a 17-year-old girl developed diarrhoea, which became more severe until she was passing 10–12 liquid stools daily with a lot of flatus. She had little constitutional upset, no abdominal pain, but 5 kg weight loss.
(a) What does microscopy of the stool show?
(b) Are the stool findings related to her symptoms?
(c) Would further investigation be helpful?
(d) Are there sequelae to this disorder?
(e) How is the disorder acquired?

4

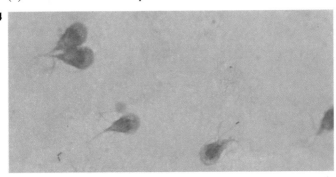

5 A young girl became vaguely ill with listlessness, loss of appetite and a low-grade fever.
(a) What can be seen on her chest X-ray?
(b) What is the probable cause?
(c) What is the nature of the lesion, and how would it evolve?
(d) How would the diagnosis be confirmed?

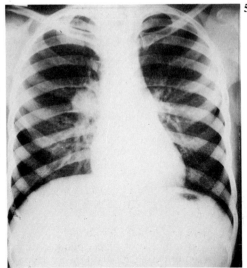

6 A young man returned to London from Zambia via Kenya. A week later, he felt unwell with intermittent pyrexia and headache and treated himself for influenza. Three days later he was behaving peculiarly and was referred to hospital.
(a) What does the peripheral blood film show?
(b) What is the basis of his abnormal behaviour?
(c) Is treatment urgent and what is the prognosis?
(d) After 48 hours of treatment, what will the blood film show?

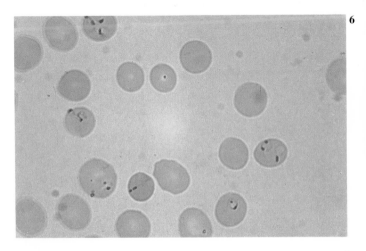

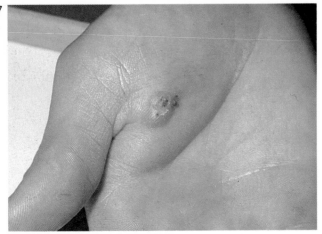

7 A young farmer noticed a painless papule on his hand. The swelling enlarged slowly over a period of 10 days but did not form a blister.
(a) What is the differential diagnosis?
(b) What is the infecting agent?
(c) What other features may appear?
(d) Will the lesion leave a scar?

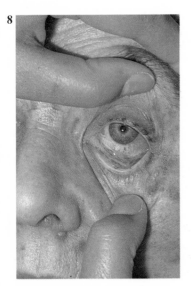

8 A woman suddenly became ill with shivering, nausea, vomiting, severe headache and a high fever. Within a few hours she developed a generalised rash, followed shortly by circulatory collapse.
(a) What can be seen in her eye?
(b) What is the nature of the rash?
(c) What is the infection?
(d) What complication is likely to have developed?
(e) What laboratory results would confirm the suspected diagnosis?

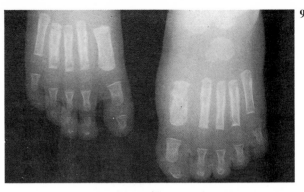

9 This 10-month-old Nigerian baby developed swelling of both feet and a high fever.
(a) What abnormality does the X-ray show?
(b) What is the name of the syndrome?
(c) Should evidence of infection be sought?
(d) Are other bony lesions likely to appear?
(e) Does the condition carry any mortality?

10 A young boy awakened with a rash on his trunk, which quickly spread to his face and limbs.
(a) Are lesions in his mouth likely?
(b) For how long does the condition remain infectious?
(c) What is the histopathology of the blisters?
(d) What are the common complications in children?

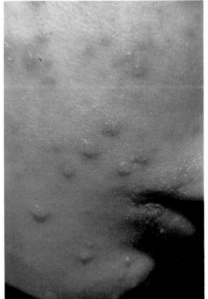

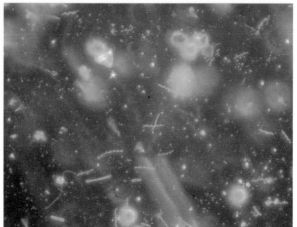

11 Five weeks after returning from 6 months in East Africa, a 28-year-old man felt unwell with a fever, and was given a 3-day course of chloroquine for presumed malaria, without improvement. The next day he developed a non-irritating, persistent rash on his trunk; 6 days ago he became jaundiced. Today his temperature is 38°C and he has some ulceration of his mouth, which has been swabbed. His alkaline phosphatase level is 4 times the upper limit of normal.
(a) What does the dark-field examination of the mouth swab show?
(b) Is the swab finding of importance?
(c) Is the rash or the jaundice caused by the course of chloroquine?
(d) Is there any effective treatment?

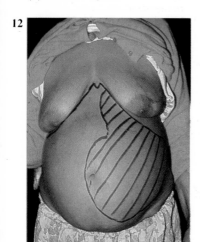

12 A 30-year-old woman from the Sudan presented with fever, abdominal discomfort and general ill-health. She was febrile and had a very large mass in the left side of her abdomen.
(a) What is the differential diagnosis?
(b) What would be the most useful single investigation?
(c) If an infective cause is demonstrated, what would her full blood count be expected to show?
(d) Would splenic aspiration be helpful?

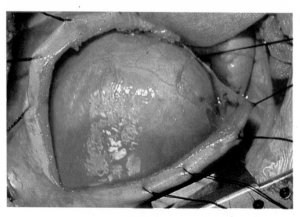

13 A girl spent the first 12 years of her life in the Sudan and Uganda. At 10 years old she suffered a sudden respiratory illness, with surgical intervention. At 20 years old she developed right upper quadrant pain. The liver, viewed from above, is shown at operation.
(a) What was the cause of the respiratory distress?
(b) Why was the second operation performed?
(c) What investigations preceded the second operation?
(d) Is she likely to have further trouble?

14 A teenage boy from Malawi had suffered haematuria for 3 weeks. It consisted of a small drop of blood at the end of micturition and had been present on most occasions. There was no frequency or dysuria.

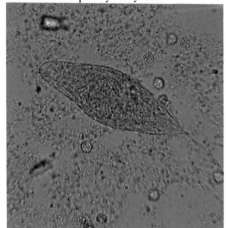

(a) What does urine microscopy show?
(b) How is the condition acquired?
(c) What is the pathogenesis of the haematuria?
(d) Is any further investigation necessary?
(e) Are there any serious complications?

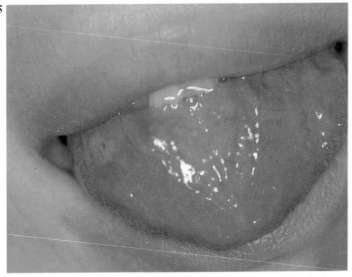

15 A child developed a mild feverish illness and complained of a painful mouth. She had a few shallow ulcers on her tongue and on her buccal mucosa. Her sister had a similar illness in the previous week.
(a) Should a skin rash be expected?
(b) What is the condition called?
(c) What is the aetiology?
(d) What differences are expected in a very young child with this disease?

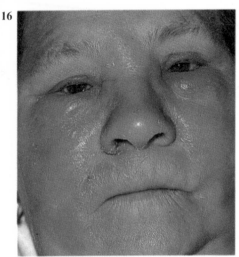

16 A woman complained of tightness and, tingling in her face, followed by a red patch which spread to both sides of her face.
(a) What is the diagnosis?
(b) What organism is responsible?
(c) Does the patient develop firm immunity?
(d) What are the common sites for this condition?

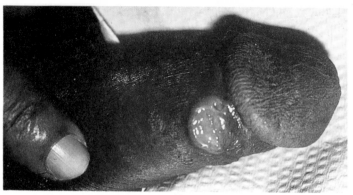

17 A 23-year-old West Indian noticed a painless sore on his penis. It is indurated but not tender and there is an enlarged non-tender gland in his left groin.
(a) What is the differential diagnosis?
(b) How may the diagnosis be confirmed?
(c) What is the natural history of an untreated lesion?
(d) Is the patient now immune to re-infection?
(e) Are there any serious sequelae?

18 A Brazilian child had been unwell for a week with fever becoming rather drowsy. She had had a swollen eye 2 weeks ago. She is now febrile (38.5°C) with marked tachycardia (140 min) and some oedema of her feet.
(a) What does the blood film show?
(b) Is the blood film finding related to the clinical features?
(c) What is the prognosis of this acute illness?
(d) Is she likely to develop long-term sequelae?
(e) Could the condition have been prevented?

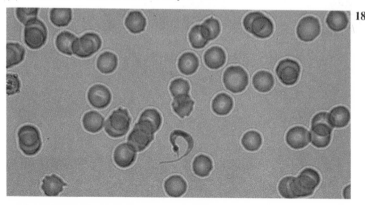

19

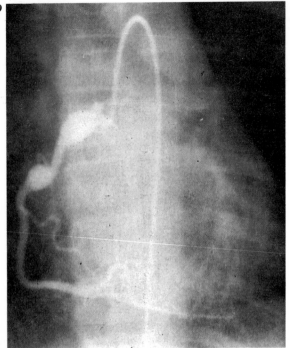

19 During convalescence after a feverish illness in a young child, a coronary arteriogram was taken.
(a) What does the arteriogram show?
(b) What disease has caused these changes?
(c) What features would be expected during the acute illness?
(d) What further complication may appear?

20 (a) What abnormality is apparent on this X-ray?
(b) What carrier state may be associated with this condition?
(c) Would operation cure the carrier state?
(d) Could chemotherapy produce a cure without operation?

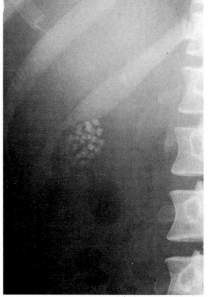

21 A baby with gastro-enteritis has a nappy rash.
(a) What is the probable cause?
(b) Where does the infection originate?
(c) What factors may contribute?

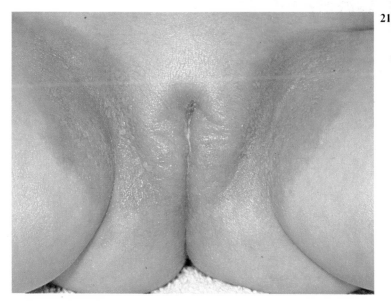

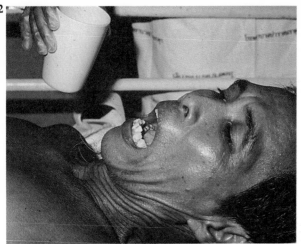

22 A patient is being offered a drink of water.
(a) What is the state he exhibits?
(b) What is the mechanism of its production?
(c) What is the aetiology?
(d) What is the prognosis?
(e) Could the disorder have been prevented?

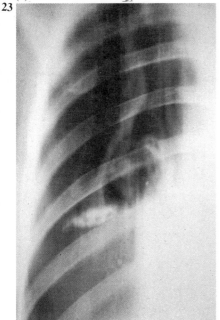

23 A woman had completed a standard course of treatment for pulmonary tuberculosis 6 months previously. Her septum was negative for acid-fast bacilli but she continued to have a productive cough with occasional haemoptysis.
(a) What is the radiological abnormality?
(b) Is further anti-tuberculosis therapy required?
(c) What is the cause of the radiological abnormality?
(d) How may the suspected diagnosis be confirmed?

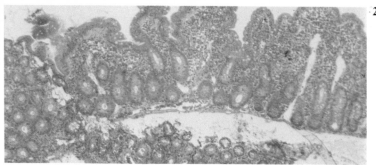

24 A young woman had been travelling in India for 12 months. During the previous 3 months she had been greatly troubled by diarrhoea and flatulence. Her appetite had remained quite good but she had lost 5 kg in weight and her energy was decreased. An infective agent was found on stool examination and a biopsy was performed. A section is shown.
(a) What tissue has been biopsied, and why?
(b) What does the biopsy show?
(c) What other investigations would be appropriate?
(d) Would an X-ray examination be helpful?
(e) What was the organism found in the stool?

25 A 5-year-old was recovering from an attack of measles when he had a convulsion. Subsequently he remained drowsy for several days, although there were no focal signs in the central nervous system.
(a) What does the electroencephalogram show?
(b) What is the cause of the disturbance?   (c) What is the prognosis?

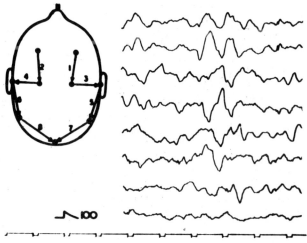

26

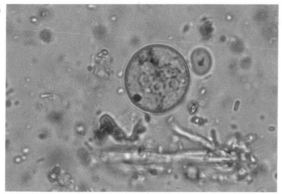

26 A 32-year-old Indian woman, living in Europe, developed diarrhoea on visiting India. It persisted two weeks after returning to Europe. Sigmoidoscopic examination is normal.
(a) What does stool microscopy show?
(b) What is the relationship between the stool findings and her symptoms?
(c) Is further investigation necessary?
(d) Is she infectious to others?
(e) Does she have amoebic colitis?

27 A skin lesion, 4 mm in diameter, became umbilicated then discharged caseous material.
(a) What is the diagnosis?   (c) What is the incubation period?
(b) What is the causative organism?   (d) How is the infection spread?

27

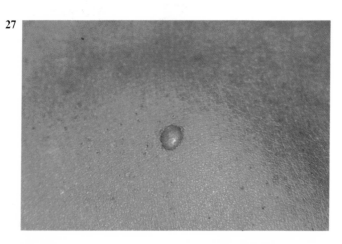

28 A 50-year-old African presented with many years' history of deformity of his lower legs and feet. His general health has been good.

(a) What does the photograph show?

(b) What is the aetiology?

(c) How was the condition acquired?

(d) How may the diagnosis be confirmed?

(e) Could the condition have been prevented?

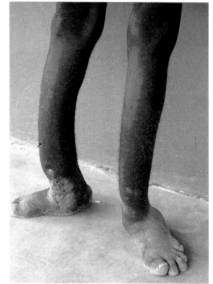

29 A shepherd suddenly became ill during lambing with fever, malaise and myalgia. He had a severe headache with retro-orbital pain and developed some neck stiffness. His cerebrospinal fluid was normal. Within a week he had a slight cough and his chest X-ray was abnormal.

(a) What is the most probable diagnosis?

(b) Is the illness related to his occupation?

(c) What is the causative organism?

(d) What is the incubation period?

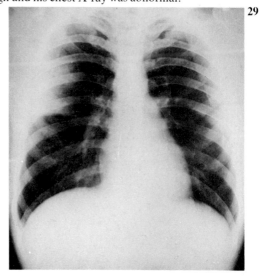

30

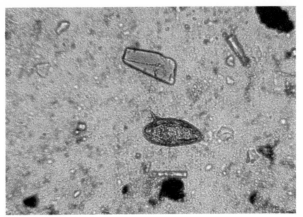

30 A 12-year-old Brazilian child presented with haematemesis. On examination the liver was palpable 2 cm below the right costal margin, and the spleen 3 cm below the left costal margin.
(a) What does stool microscopy show?
(b) What is the origin of the stool finding?
(c) Are the symptoms and stool findings related?
(d) What is the pathogenesis of the haematemesis?
(e) What is the prognosis?

31

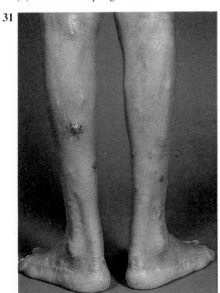

31 A man developed bluish-red macules and papules on his legs. The lesions became heavily pigmented.
(a) What is the condition?
(b) How would you confirm the diagnosis?
(c) With what infection may it be associated?
(d) What other organs may be involved?

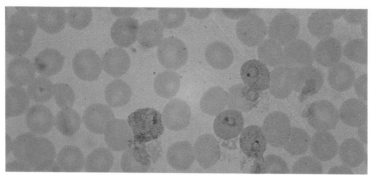

32 For 2 years a 35-year-old man was working in Papua, New Guinea, where he suffered febrile attacks, which were treated as malaria; blood films were not examined. Two months ago he returned to Britain, and 2 days ago had an attack of fever. Yesterday he felt better but today feels unwell: temperature 38.6°C.
(a) What does the peripheral blood film show?
(b) Is there anything unusual about the abnormality present?
(c) Could this febrile attack be part of the illness he suffered abroad?
(d) Will a course of schizontocide be curative?
(e) What are the sequelae of this condition?

33 A child aged 2 years had a convulsion at the onset of a feverish illness; he had an inflamed throat but no exudate. After 4 days the fever settled and an erythematous macular rash appeared. This persisted for only 36 hours. A throat swab was negative for *Streptococcus pyogenes* and a white blood cell count was normal.
(a) What is the most probable diagnosis?
(b) What is the cause?
(c) What is the incubation period?
(d) What is the most common complication?

34 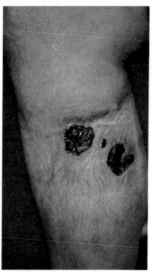 **34** A 32-year-old man had been working in Nigeria for 2 years. Three months ago he developed a lesion on the inner surface of his leg just below his knee. Treatment did not help, and the fairly painless lesion increased in size. It appeared to be superficial, causing no constitutional upset.

(a) What is the diagnosis?

(b) Will it spread to involve deeper structures, including bone?

(c) In the absence of effective treatment, will the lesion extend to involve a progressively larger area?

(d) Is discharge a feature of the lesion?

(e) How may a firm diagnosis be made?

35 A child developed a unilateral mucopurulent conjunctivitis 10 days after birth. A conjunctival smear was stained by Giemsa's method.

(a) What does the smear show?

(b) What is the diagnosis?

(c) What is the causative organism?

(d) What complications may develop?

35

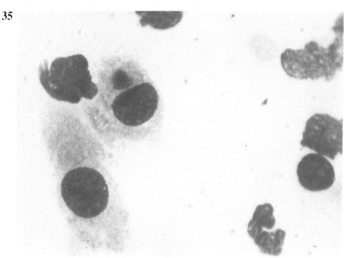

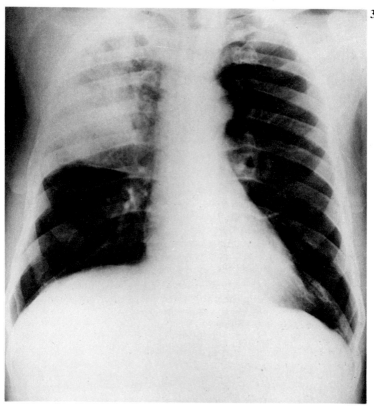

36 A 67-year-old man was admitted to hospital for treatment of chronic lymphatic leukaemia. A week after discharge he developed a flu-like illness with a dry cough, then felt nauseated and had watery diarrhoea. His breathing became progressively more distressed with a pleuritic type of pain in the right side of his chest. Within 4 days he was gravely ill with a continuous high fever and was somnolent and very confused. Investigations showed: WBC $8.2 \times 10^9/1$, ESR 90 mm in 1 hour, serum Na^+ 121 mmol/1, serum bilirubin 40 μmol/1, serum aspartate transaminase 45 U/1, serum albumin 24 g/l.

(a) What does the chest X-ray show?
(b) What is the probable diagnosis?
(c) How would you confirm the diagnosis?
(d) Is this likely to be a nosocomial infection?
(e) What is the probable source of the infection?

37

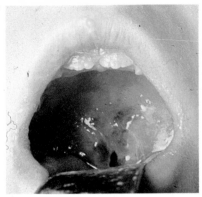

37 A young girl became vaguely off-colour, with loss of appetite and listlessness but no fever. By the end of a week she was gravely ill with waxy pallor, extreme lassitude and drowsiness. She later developed circulatory failure and died.

(a) What does the photograph show?

(b) What is the diagnosis?

(c) What is the case of the circulatory failure?

(d) If she had survived the acute stage, what other complications may have developed?

38 A 9-year-old boy fell under a tractor in a farmyard and sustained a penetrating wound of the thigh. There was some delay before obtaining medical attention and 48 hours elapsed before the wound was explored and necrotic tissue and clothing removed.

(a) What does the swab culture show, and how was it cultured?

(b) What was the source of this organism?

(c) Is the finding of importance?

(d) Is any additional treatment indicated?

(e) What is the prognosis?

38

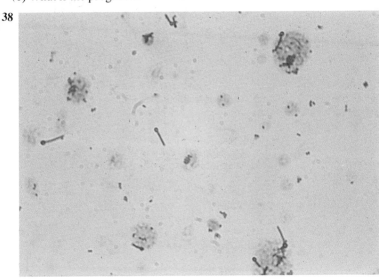

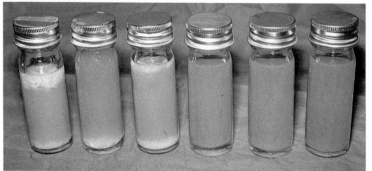

39 An 18-year-old girl had lived in Uganda and the Sudan from birth to aged 10. She presented with abdominal discomfort in the right hypochondrium; ultrasonic scanning showed a space-occupying lesion in the right lobe of the liver. At operation a mass was found in the liver which, on aspiration, produced the material shown.
(a) What was responsible for the lesion in the liver?
(b) What would microscopic examination of the material show?
(c) Should the lesion be removed?
(d) Are there dangers in removing it?
(e) Is the liver lesion likely to recur?

40 A nurse had a routine chest X-ray. She was well and had no history of serious illness apart from measles, varicella and pertussis. She resided in the UK and had not travelled abroad.
(a) What is apparent on the X-ray plate?
(b) What is the most probable cause of the condition?
(c) What is the pathology?
(d) What is the prognosis?

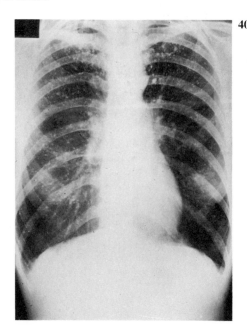

41

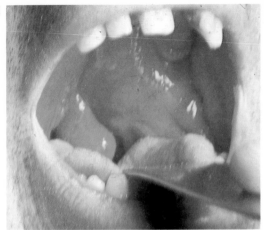

41 A man became ill with a sore throat. A few days later he had difficulty in swallowing and had developed a nasal intonation to his voice.
(a) What is the diagnosis?
(b) What is the natural course of the illness?
(c) What organisms may be responsible?
(d) What underlying condition may be present?

42 A patient with herpes zoster affecting the forehead complained of poor vision.
(a) What is the diagnosis?
(b) Why is the pupil irregular?
(c) What other sign would point to the possibility of this complication?
(d) What precaution should be taken to limit the extent of the damage?

42

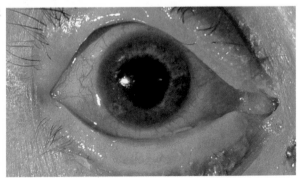

43 These virus particles were found by electron microscopy in the stool of a young child with gastro-enteritis.
(a) What is the virus?
(b) What are the presenting features of the illness?
(c) How common is this infection in a developed country?
(d) How frequently do adults become ill with this infection?

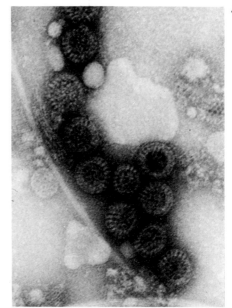

44 A woman from a tropical Pacific island had a widespread scaly eruption, which spread to her scalp, palms of her hands and soles of her feet. She had no constitutional disturbance.
(a) What is the differential diagnosis?
(b) What is the causative organism?
(c) What are the predisposing causes?

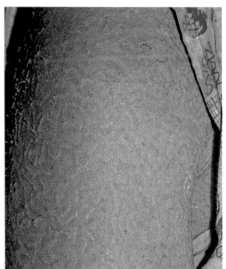

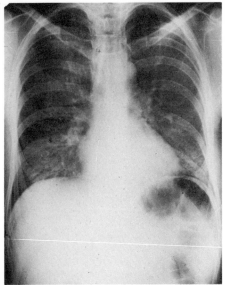

45 A young man had persistent enlargement of his lymph nodes, chronic candidiasis of his mouth and intermittent bouts of diarrhoea. He then developed a cough and became progressively more breathless.
(a) What does the chest X-ray show?
(b) What is the probable cause of the respiratory symptoms?
(c) What is the underlying disease?
(d) How could the nature of the lung infection be confirmed?
(e) What is the primary infectious agent?

46 A 28-year-old man has been working in tropical Africa for the past 3 years. One week ago he developed pyrexia and a pain in the left groin. Over the next 2 days his left leg became inflamed and painful, and a tender lump appeared in his groin.
(a) What does the peripheral blood film show?
(b) How is the condition acquired?
(c) What is the pathogenesis of the illness?
(d) Are there other features of the condition?
(e) What is the prognosis?

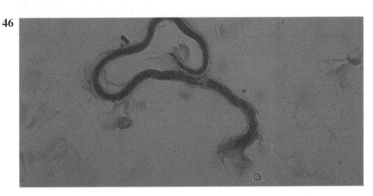

47 (a) What eye defect is shown?
(b) What is the cause?
(c) What is the prognosis?

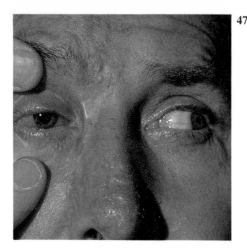

48 A 12-year-old Iranian boy noticed painless sores on his nose and cheek for about 6 weeks. They had gradually increased in size. The rest of his skin was clear and there was no constitutional upset.
(a) What is the most probable infective diagnosis?
(b) What is the means of transmission?
(c) How is the diagnosis confirmed?
(d) Is generalised infection a danger?
(e) What is the prognosis if untreated?

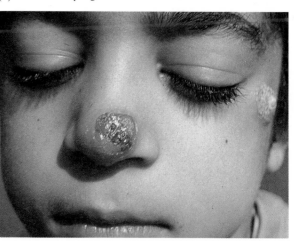

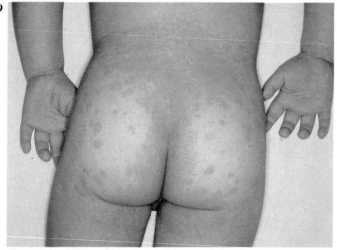

49 A Japanese boy became ill with a high fever accompanied by conjunctivitis, an erythematous rash, induration of the dorsum of his hands and feet, stomatitis with a strawberry tongue and enlargement of the lymph nodes in his neck. He remained ill despite antibiotic therapy; routine investigations proved to be negative.
(a) What is the probable diagnosis?
(b) What other physical sign may appear to support the diagnosis?
(c) What life-threatening complication may develop?
(d) What is the usual platelet count in this disease?

50 (a) What is the diagnosis?
(b) What organisms cause this disease?
(c) How does the infection arise, and what structures are involved?

50

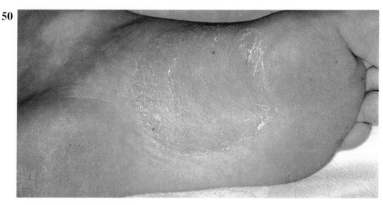

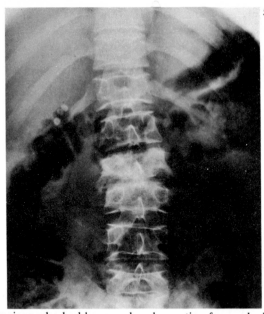

51 A 22-year-old Jamaican who had been under observation for marked anaemia for 20 years, presented with a short history of back pain.
(a) What does the radiograph show?
(b) What is the probable aetiology?
(c) What is the relationship between the X-ray appearance and his anaemia?
(d) Are these conditions common in patients with this basic abnormality?
(e) What is the prognosis?

52 A virus was detected on electron microscopy of fluid from a vesicle on the skin of a child.

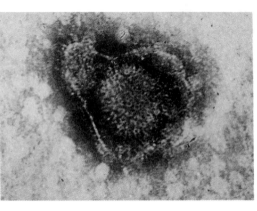

(a) To what group of viruses does it belong?
(b) Does it contain DNA or RNA?
(c) Name 4 common diseases of man caused by these viruses.
(d) What is the most probable diagnosis in a child?

53

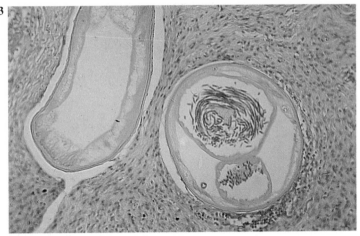

53 Eight years ago, a 28-year-old man from West Africa was given tablets for a skin irritation. Since then it has recurred intermittently, particularly severely over the past few months. There is a maculopapular rash over his buttocks and lower legs, and two small nodules in the region of the iliac crests.
(a) What does the section of the nodule show?
(b) Are the section findings related to the clinical features?
(c) Can a diagnosis be made in the absence of nodules?
(d) What is the pathogenesis of the disorder?
(e) Are there other serious features of the condition?

54

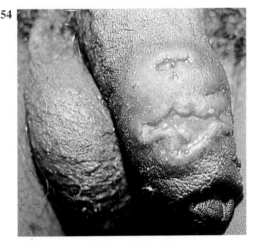

54 A 28-year-old man from a poor West African city presented with ulceration of the penile shaft, which started as a painful swelling 6 days previously. The ulceration area is tender but not indurated, and a lymph node in one groin is also tender.
(a) What is the most probable diagnosis?
(b) How may the diagnosis be confirmed?
(c) Should any other investigation be made?
(d) Are there any serious complications?

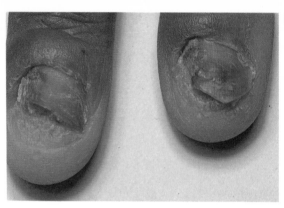

55 A 35-year-old kitchen worker presented with a 2-year history of deformity of the finger-nails, for which much treatment was given. There has been no constitutional upset and the rest of the clinical examination was normal.
(a) What is the differential diagnosis?
(b) How may the diagnosis be confirmed?
(c) Are there any factors predisposing to this condition?
(d) What is the natural history of the condition?
(e) What is the prognosis?

56 An old lady developed a painful rash on her forehead and side of her nose.
(a) What is the primary disease?
(b) What is the eye complication?
(c) What is the prognosis of the eye condition?
(d) Would she have any persistent disturbance of her cornea?

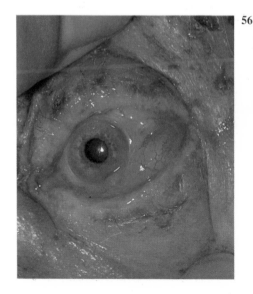

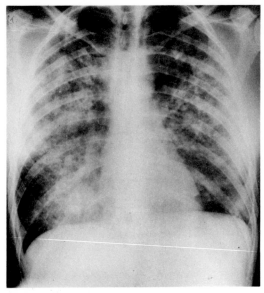

57 Four days after the onset of an attack of varicella a young man developed a cough. His condition rapidly deteriorated and he became breathless and markedly cyanosed.

(a) What does the X-ray film show?
(b) What is the aetiology?
(c) What is the histopathology?
(d) Is this condition found in children with varicella?

58 A man developed an itchy papule on the side of his neck, followed by a cluster of haemorrhagic vesicles. The central area dried up to form a thick leathery dark scab. The lesion was painless.
(a) What is the diagnosis?
(b) What is his occupation?
(c) What organism is responsible?
(d) What would be his white blood cell count?
(e) Can the infection be transmitted from man to man?

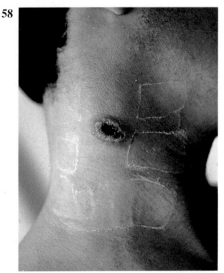

59 A man developed a feverish illness with a cough. Within a week a rash appeared on his trunk. The individual lesions blanched on pressure. The white blood cell count was 4.5 × 10⁹/l with a neutropenia.

(a) What is the probable diagnosis?
(b) What is the rash called?
(c) What is the most reliable method of confirming the diagnosis?
(d) What are the two most important complications?

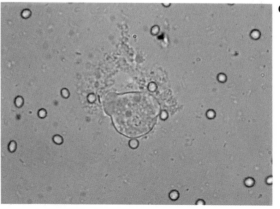

60 A young European had been in India for 3 months. Ten days ago she developed diarrhoea, 6 days ago she noticed blood in her stools. She had little constitutional upset and only mild lower-abdominal pain. Sigmoidoscopy showed small discrete mucosal ulcers separated by mucosa, which was not greatly inflamed.

(a) What does the stool microscopy show?
(b) Is any further investigation needed to determine the cause of this disorder?
(c) If untreated, what is the natural history of this disorder?
(d) After recovery, are there likely to be any sequelae?
(e) How is the condition acquired?

61

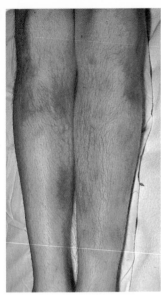

61 A young woman complained of tender swellings on her legs. Two weeks previously she had an attack of diarrhoea, accompanied by abdominal pain.
(a) What is the rash on her legs?
(b) What is the probable cause of her intestinal upset?
(c) Would a rash be expected elsewhere?
(d) How long would the rash persist?

62 A 30-year-old woman lived in Belgium until 11 months ago, when she went to Central America to study bats in caves. Twelve days ago she developed an acute respiratory illness with pyrexia, persistent non-productive cough and shortness of breath.

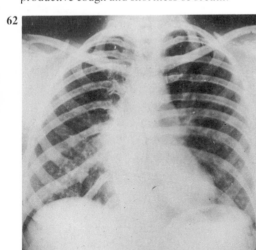

(a) What does the radiograph show?
(b) What is the differential diagnosis?
(c) How may the diagnosis be confirmed?
(d) What is the prognosis?
(e) Will the X-ray appearance change?

63 A man had recurrent attacks of blisters on his penis.
(a) What is the diagnosis?
(b) What virus is responsible?
(c) Name two neurological complications of this type of infection.
(d) Are infections with this virus usually symptomatic in the male?

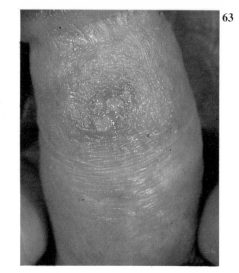

64 A young man became ill with fever, headache and sore throat. He had a generalised non-itchy maculopapular rash and generalised enlargement of his lymph nodes. His throat was inflamed but there was no exudate. The rash persisted for 5 weeks.
(a) What is the most probable diagnosis?
(b) What other clinical evidence would support the diagnosis?
(c) Is the condition infectious?
(d) How could the diagnosis be confirmed?

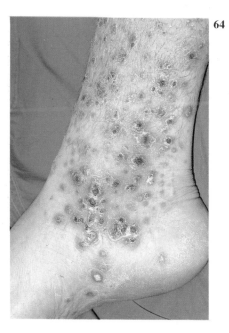

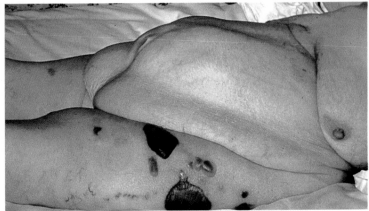

65 An elderly woman became gravely ill following operation on a strangulated femoral hernia. She complained of severe pain in her thigh and became profoundly shocked.
(a) What is the probable diagnosis?
(b) What is the commonest organism causing this condition?
(c) What would X-ray examination of the affected area show?
(d) What complication may develop?

66 A West African child presented with a swollen hand, on which there were multiple skin lesions. There were skin lesions elsewhere, but little constitutional upset.
(a) What is the diagnosis?
(b) What would X-ray examination of the hand show?
(c) What would be the result of blood culture?
(d) Should the child be isolated?
(e) How would the diagnosis be confirmed?

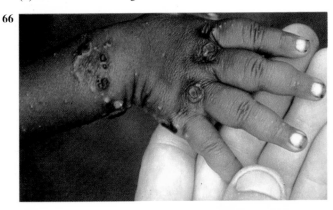

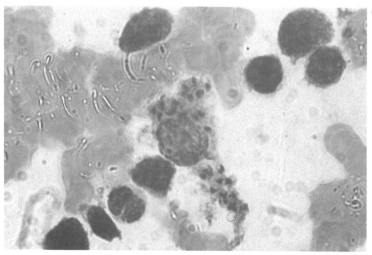

67 A young man lived in Aden for 1 year. Four weeks ago he became unwell with a fever, which varied from day to day and was accompanied by sweats. He was febrile and his spleen was just palpable. Blood cultures remained sterile over the first week. His haemoglobin level was 12.4 g/dl, his white blood cell count 3.6 × 10⁹/l and his platelet count 130 × 10⁹/l. Bone marrow aspirate is shown.
(a) What is the differential diagnosis?
(b) Has the diagnosis been established?
(c) What other means are available for making the diagnosis?
(d) Is treatment necessary?

68 A child dev-
eloped a rash on
his buttock.
(a) What is the
diagnosis?
(b) Is this a
primary attack?
(c) What or-
ganism is respon-
sible?
(d) What other
condition may be
mistaken for this
eruption?

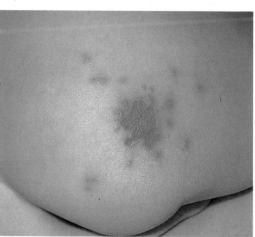

69

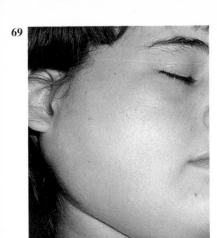

69 A young girl had an appendicectomy. Postoperatively she became feverish and developed painful swelling of her face. A white blood cell count showed a marked polymorphonuclear leucocytosis.
(a) What is the nature of the swelling?
(b) What clinical signs may be present?
(c) What are the predisposing causes?
(d) What organism is likely to cause this condition?

70 A 16-year-old girl from Ethiopia and the Sudan experienced mild right upper quadrant discomfort over the past few months. She has now become acutely ill with rigors and a high fever. Her liver is enlarged and tender but there is no definite jaundice.
(a) What does the ultrasonic scan of the liver show?
(b) What is the differential diagnosis?
(c) How would the diagnosis be confirmed?
(d) What complications may develop?

70

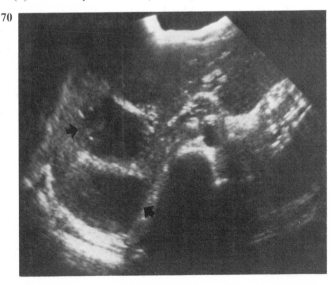

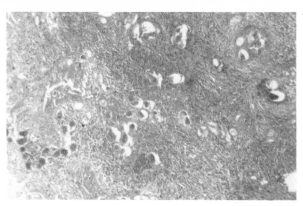

71 A 28-year-old man from Iraq gave a history of having had haematuria for several weeks up to 1 month ago. He had it as a child and at 18-years-old, and was treated both times. No abnormality was found in his urine on microscopy or culture. An intravenous pyelogram showed minor dilatation of one renal pelvis; cystoscopy was carried out and biopsy performed.
(a) What is the differential diagnosis of haematuria in this patient?
(b) What possible cause has been excluded so far?
(c) What does the bladder biopsy show?
(d) What is the pathogenesis of the haematuria?
(e) May complete recovery be obtained?

72 A teenage boy with an exudative tonsillitis was treated with ampicillin. It did not respond and after a few days he developed a generalised rash.
(a) What is the diagnosis?
(b) How would the diagnosis be confirmed?
(c) How common is the rash in these circumstances?

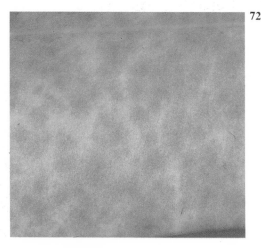

73

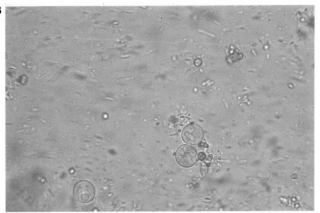

73 A 26-year-old Venezuelan man complained of having had skin irritation for 6 months.
(a) What does his stool microscopy show?
(b) Are the stool findings and the symptoms related?
(c) Does the patient need treatment?
(d) If he is not treated, will the stool findings alter?
(e) Is the patient a public health risk?

74 A patient had intermittent bouts of fever with weight loss and progressive anaemia.
(a) What is the physical sign?
(b) What is the underlying disease?
(c) What is the cause of the sign?
(d) What other signs may be detected?

74

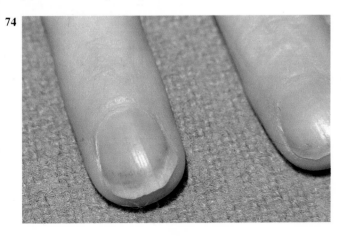

75 A 27-year-old West African gave a 5-year history of weakness and deformity of his hands. Recently he developed swelling of his face and nodules on the arms and legs. He had pale, flat, poorly demarcated lesions on his trunk.

(a) What is the most probable diagnosis?

(b) Has the form of his illness altered?

(c) What are the nodules on his limbs and swellings of his face?

(d) How may the diagnosis be established?

(e) Should the patient be isolated?

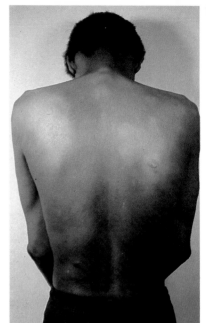

76 (a) What is the diagnosis?

(b) What is the causative organism?

(c) What are the common sites of this infection?

(d) What is the source of the infection?

(e) What complications may develop?

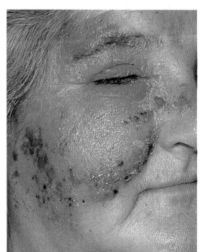

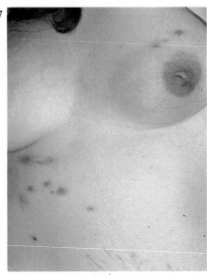

77 A woman became ill about 3 weeks after returning home from hospital following the birth of her baby.
(a) From what is she suffering?
(b) What is the most probable infecting agent?
(c) What is the immediate source of infection?
(d) What is the public health significance of this infection?

78 A young woman, who suffered from eczema, became ill with a high fever and developed a vesicular rash, most severe in those areas of her skin affected by the eczema.
(a) What is the diagnosis?
(b) How would the diagnosis be confirmed?
(c) How is the infection spread?
(d) Are other organs affected?

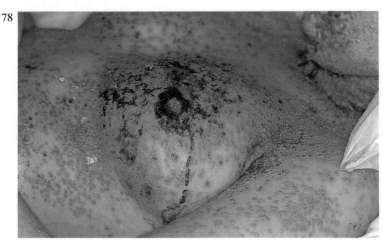

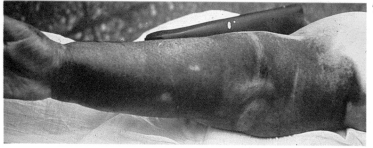

79 An Iraqi woman suddenly became ill, with a high fever, headache and severe pains in her limbs and back. Her face and neck became oedematous, and her conjunctivae and pharynx were injected. After 2 days small haemorrhages were seen on her palate and a fine petechial rash appeared on her back, spreading to cover her entire body. On the 5th day there was extensive extravasation of blood into the subcutaneous tissues.
(a) What is the probable diagnosis?
(b) What is the likely cause?
(c) How is the infection transmitted?
(d) What is the reservoir of infection?

80 (a) What does this radiograph show?
(b) What is the commonest known infectious cause?
(c) What other conditions may be present?
(d) When a pregnant mother has a primary infection, what is the risk to her baby?

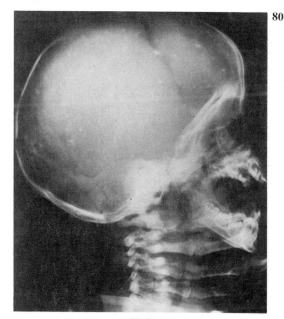

81

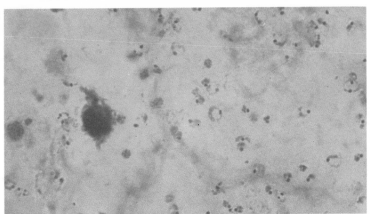

81 A 60-year-old American woman was in Kenya for 3 weeks. Four days ago she felt unwell with pyrexia and headache which persisted. Her blood urea is 30 mmol/1.
(a) What does the peripheral thick blood film show?
(b) What is the parasitaemia?
(c) Is the blood urea value of importance?
(d) What is the prognosis?

82 A young adult became ill with a painful mouth and mild constitutional disturbance.
(a) What is the differential diagnosis?
(b) Is the infection likely to be primary or recurrent?
(c) How could the diagnosis be confirmed?
(d) Which virus is likely to cause the disease?

82

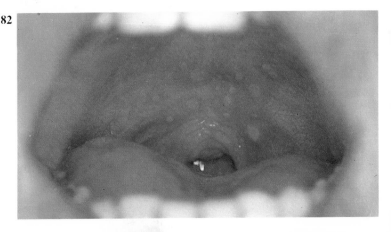

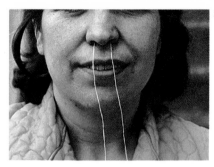

83 A 40-year-old South American woman complained of blood-stained nasal discharge. She had been treated for this some years previously. There was no constitutional upset. Her nasal septum was perforated and there was a healed scar on her wrist.
(a) What infections may result in perforation of the nasal septum?
(b) What is the significance of the scar on her wrist?
(c) What investigations are indicated?
(d) How may the diagnosis be established with certainty?
(e) What is the prognosis?

84 (a) What is the lesion?
(b) What organism is responsible?
(c) Name a predisposing cause.
(d) What is the pathology?

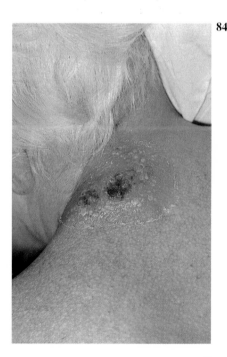

85

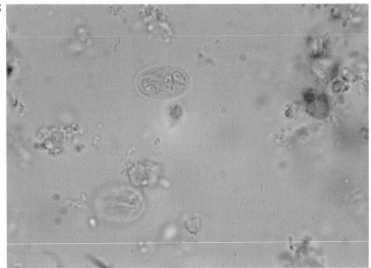

85 A 35-year-old Englishman had been in India for 6 weeks where he had two attacks of diarrhoea and once passed a little blood. Four years ago he had diarrhoea with blood in his stool and was treated for three months. He returned from India two days ago, with continuing diarrhoea. Today sigmoidoscopy shows a somewhat inflamed rectum with contact bleeding.

(a) What does stool microscopy show?

(b) What is the relationship between the current illness and the stool finding?

(c) Would any other investigation be helpful?

(d) What is the most likely diagnosis today?

(e) What is the prognosis?

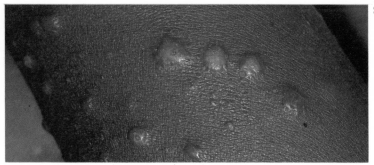

86 A girl developed varicella while on holiday in Grenada, West Indies. The pustules were unusually large and she became oliguric, with protein and blood in her urine.
(a) What is the complication?
(b) What other features would be expected?
(c) What organism is responsible for the complication?
(d) Is the visit to the tropics relevant?
(e) What is the prognosis?

87 A 30-year-old man presented with a 1-year history of discharging lesions on the upper neck and back. There had been some constitutional upset.
(a) What is the diagnosis?
(b) How is the condition acquired?
(c) Is macroscopic examination of the discharge helpful?
(d) How may the diagnosis be confirmed?
(e) Is the chest X-ray likely to be abnormal?

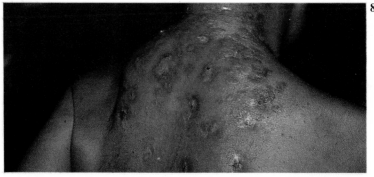

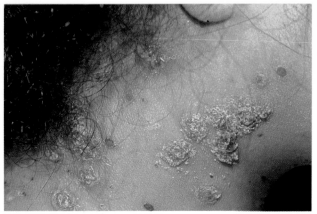

88 (a) What is the skin infection?
(b) What is the causative organism?
(c) What underlying conditions may be present?

89 A young girl suddenly became ill with chills followed by a sharp rise in temperature. She complained of severe headache, myalgia and weakness. After 4 days she developed a generalised rash with a haemorrhagic element and a migratory arthritis. Her white blood cell count showed a marked polymorphonuclear leucocytosis. After several days her temperature fell by crisis but subsequently rose again.
(a) What is the differential diagnosis?
(b) What is the probable diagnosis?
(c) What is the causative organism?
(d) How is it transmitted?
(e) What is the natural course of the illness?

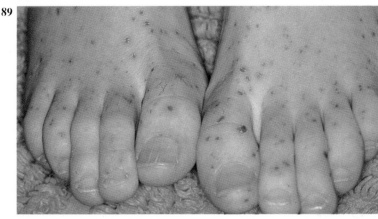

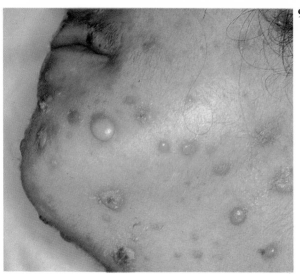

90 A woman with Hodgkin's disease developed a vesicular rash which became pustular. The lesions came out in crops and had a generalised distribution, although the rash was heavier on the central areas of the body. She continued to run a high fever and became jaundiced.
(a) What is the diagnosis of the rash?
(b) What investigation is essential to determine the cause of the fever?
(c) What are the possible causes of the jaundice?
(d) What is the prognosis?

91 A woman became ill with a high fever and developed a generalised rash, most prominent on her limbs.
(a) What is the nature of the rash?
(b) What other features may be present?
(c) What is the cause?
(d) What is the natural course of the illness?

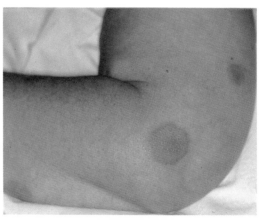

92

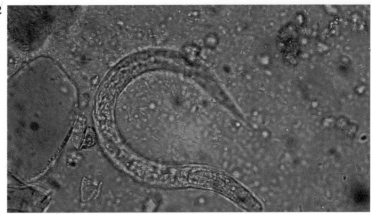

92 A 40-year-old man, who lived mainly in the humid tropics, is under treatment for lymphoma. Two weeks ago he developed diarrhoea and a cough. Chest X-ray showed soft miliary mottling.
(a) What does stool microscopy show?
(b) Is there a relationship between the stool findings and his symptoms?
(c) How is the bowel condition acquired?
(d) Why does this particular patient have these symptoms?
(e) What is the prognosis?

93 A young boy was feverish and had an acute respiratory tract infection. After 4 days a rash appeared behind his ears and spread over his face and downwards to his trunk.
(a) What is the diagnosis?
(b) What would you expect to find on examining his buccal cavity?
(c) What is the causative organism?
(d) Name two common complications.

93

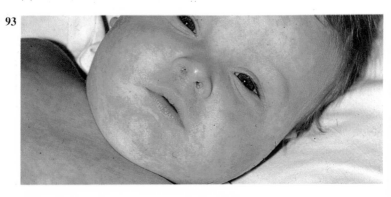

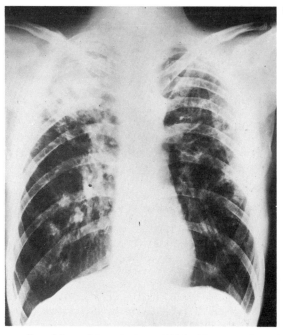

94 An elderly man suffered from 'chronic bronchitis' with a cough and shortness of breath.
(a) What does the chest X-ray show?
(b) Is the patient infectious?
(c) What organisms may be present?

95 A 17-year-old West Indian girl presented with diarrhoea lasting for 2 days, associated with abdominal cramps and low fever. The left lower quadrant of her abdomen was tender.

(a) What abnormality is apparent?
(b) Is this abnormality related to her current symptoms?
(c) What investigations should be performed?
(d) How was the oral abnormality acquired?
(e) Is the oral abnormality the only manifestation of this condition?

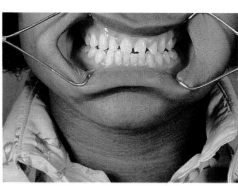

96

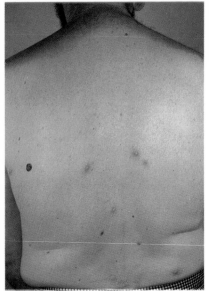

96 An archaeologist, working in a rural area of the Middle East for 6 months, developed multiple skin lesions, especially on his trunk. They were neither painful nor itchy. No constitutional upset.

(a) What is the diagnosis?

(b) What is the epidemiology?

(c) How may the diagnosis be confirmed?

(d) If untreated, what is the prognosis?

97 An 8-year-old East African boy had a haemoglobin concentration of 7 g/dl with MCV of 72 fl, and absolute eosinophil count of 1×10^9/l and reticulocyte count of 0.2 per cent.

(a) What does stool microscopy show?

(b) Are the stool and haematological findings related?

(c) Does the cause of the stool findings need to be treated?

(d) Could the anaemia be corrected without reference to the stool findings?

(e) What is the pathogenesis of the boy's anaemia?

97

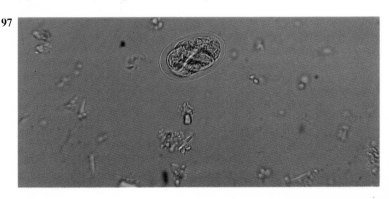

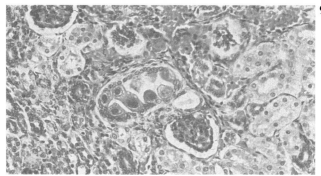

98 (a) What abnormality is present in this section of kidney?
(b) What virus is responsible?
(c) What syndromes are associated with congenital or perinatal infection?
(d) What is the relevance of the virus in transplant surgery?
(e) How is the virus transmitted to patients undergoing open-heart surgery?

99 A girl had an attack of varicella. Three days after the onset she complained of pain in her chest and was found to have a cellulitis.
(a) What has happened?
(b) What organism is likely to have caused the problem?
(c) What other acute complication may be present?
(d) What is the prognosis?

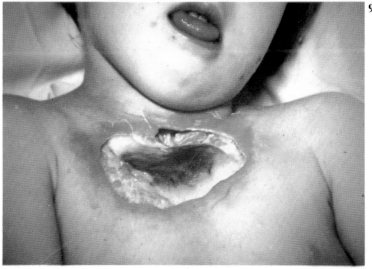

100

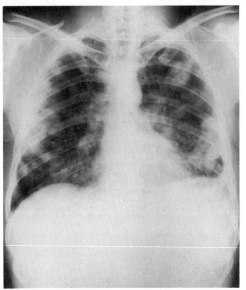

100 A 35-year-old Syrian man gave a history of bilateral pleuritic chest pain and a cough, which was mainly unproductive, although twice he had noticed a little blood in mucoid sputum. Otherwise well with no previous serious ill-health.
(a) What does the radiograph show?
(b) Is there a possible infective cause for the X-ray findings?
(c) How may the suspected cause be confirmed?
(d) What is the pathogenesis?
(e) What is the prognosis?

101 A 28-year-old British girl spent 2 years in Uganda returning home 18 months ago and remaining in Europe. She was generally well in Uganda apart from occasional diarrhoea. A week ago she developed pyrexia, which has persisted intermittently.
(a) What does the blood film show?
(b) What would be the expected pattern of the pyrexia?
(c) Is it surprising that she was well in Uganda and in Britain until now?
(d) What would a schizontocide be expected to do?
(e) What are the sequelae of this condition?

101

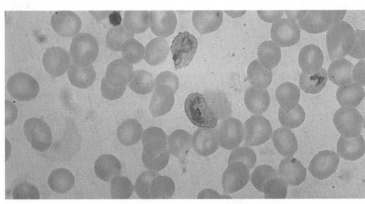

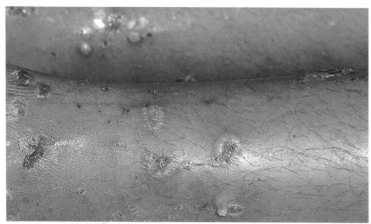

102 A girl living in the West Indies, developed a rash on her legs.
(a) What is the nature of the rash?
(b) What is the causative organism?
(c) What age groups have the highest incidence?
(d) What are the predisposing causes?
(e) What complication may develop?

103 On returning to London after sea-swimming and beach-sunbathing in the Caribbean, a young man developed an itchy rash on his trunk.
(a) What is the diagnosis?
(b) What is the cause?
(c) What is the source of the infection?

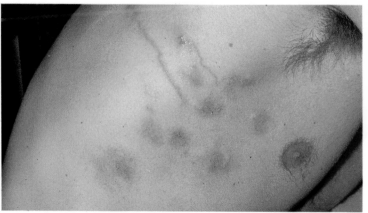

104

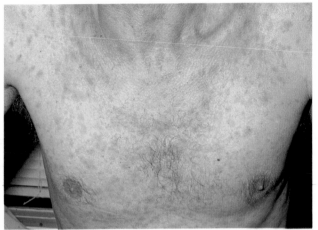

104 A young man presented with a feverish illness associated with a symmetrical generalised rash. He was found to have painless shallow ulcers in his mouth and generalised enlargement of his lymph nodes.
(a) What is the most probable diagnosis?
(b) How would the diagnosis be confirmed?
(c) Is the patient infectious?
(d) How long will the skin lesions and lymphadenopathy persist in untreated cases?

105 (a) What is the clinical diagnosis?
(b) What organisms may be responsible?
(c) Which type of infection is most likely in a child?
(d) How would the diagnosis be confirmed?

105

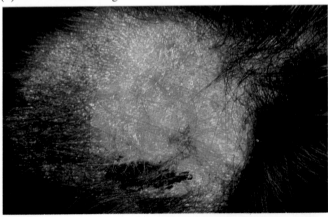

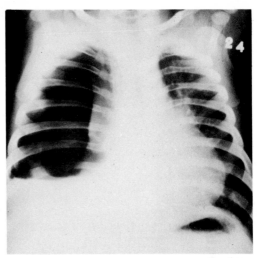

106 A boy, known to have mucoviscidosis, developed an upper respiratory infection with fever, nasal discharge and coughing. The illness progressed rapidly, with increasing respiratory distress, subcostal recession and cyanosis.
(a) What does the X-ray of his chest show?
(b) What is the diagnosis?
(c) What is the causative organism?
(d) What are the predisposing causes?

107 A 30-year-old man had been in India for the past year. A month ago he became ill with pyrexia, pain in the right side of his chest on breathing deeply, and coughing. A tender mass was found in the right upper quadrant. There was no jaundice. His white blood cell count was 14×10^9/l.
(a) What is the differential diagnosis?
(b) Would a chest X-ray be helpful?
(c) What would be the appropriate investigations?
(d) Would stool examination make a definitive diagnosis?
(e) What organism is responsible?

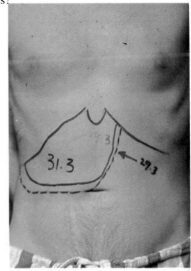

108

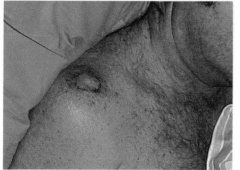

108 A 40-year-old man had been game hunting for several months in Central Africa. Ten days ago he noticed a sore on his shoulder. It increased in size, accompanied by pyrexia and malaise. There was an enlarged supraclavicular lymph node.

(a) What is the most probable diagnosis?
(b) How is the condition acquired?
(c) What would biopsy of the lesion show?
(d) How may the diagnosis be established?
(e) What is the prognosis?

109 An 18-year-old girl from southern Nigeria developed an uncomfortable swelling just above the right wrist, which restricted wrist movement. She had a similar swelling of one cheek about 6-months ago.
(a) What does the peripheral blood film show?
(b) How is the condition acquired?
(c) What other symptoms might the patient report?
(d) Do all patients with this condition show this blood film finding?
(e) What is the prognosis?

109

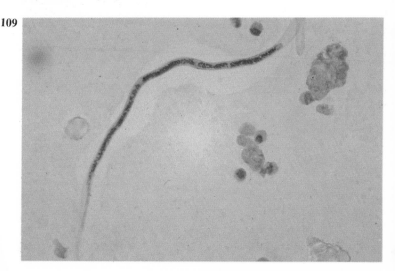

110 A boy aged 9 years was bitten on the leg by a dog 6 weeks previously; the wound healed normally but 3 days ago he became apathetic, refused food, found difficulty in walking, had neck stiffness and weakness of the lower limbs. The cerebrospinal fluid was normal.
(a) What is the diagnosis?
(b) Is the presentation atypical?
(c) How may the diagnosis be established?
(d) What is the prognosis?
(e) Can treatment influence the outcome?

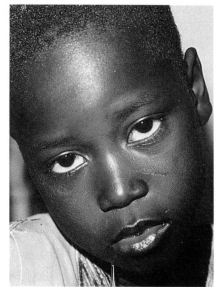

111 A girl became ill with a fever, sore throat and vomiting. Next day she developed a generalised erythematous rash. Her tongue is shown on the fifth day of her illness.
(a) What is illustrated?
(b) What is the diagnosis?
(c) Name two important complications which appear during late convalescence.
(d) What organism is responsible?

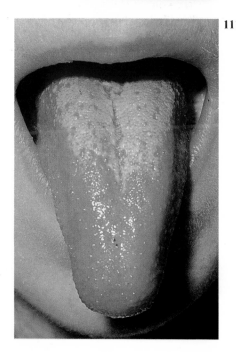

112 A Pakistani became ill with general malaise, anorexia and loss of weight, accompanied by irregular pyrexia.

(a) What does the chest X-ray show?

(b) What is the most probable diagnosis?

(c) How could the diagnosis be confirmed?

(d) What other features may be present?

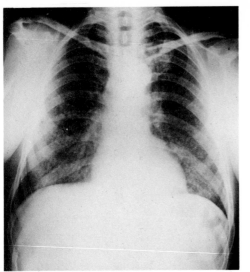

113 This week-old baby was born at home in the rural tropics. Yesterday she failed to suck and today was noticed to adopt this position occasionally.

(a) What is the condition?

(b) How is it acquired?

(c) Could it have been prevented?

(d) Is there any treatment?

(e) What is the prognosis?

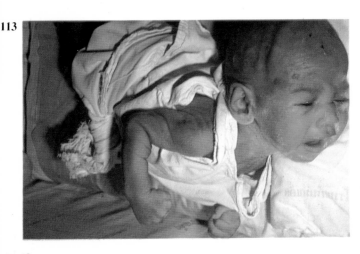

114 A woman living in England has not travelled outside Europe. During the past 5 years she has had four attacks of feverish illness associated with redness and painful swelling of her leg.
(a) What is the diagnosis?
(b) What is the causative organism?
(c) What are the predisposing factors?
(d) What complications may develop?

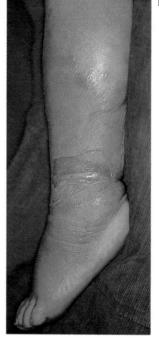

115 A young boy became feverish and developed a vesicular rash on his fingers and toes. Several shallow ulcers were found in his mouth.
(a) What is the diagnosis?
(b) What are the causative organisms?
(c) Are the skin lesions painful?
(d) How infectious is the disease?

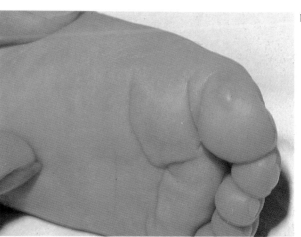

116 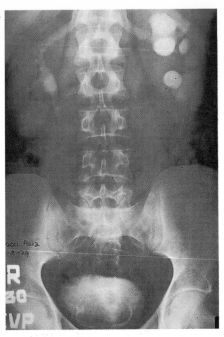 This Iraqi man aged 35 years gave a 2 year history of frequency of micturition and also intermittent haematuria 10 years previously. Recently, urine culture was sterile and an intravenous pyelogram was carried out.

(a) What does the X-ray show?

(b) Would further urine examination be helpful?

(c) If further urine examination were not helpful, what other investigations might be made?

(d) What is the pathogenesis of this condition?

(e) How is the condition acquired?

117 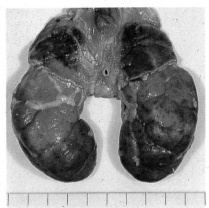 A healthy boy suddenly became ill with a high fever. Within hours an extensive haemorrhagic rash appeared on his skin and mucosae. Shortly afterwards he developed circulatory failure and died.

(a) What organs have been removed at autopsy?

(b) What abnormality is present?

(c) What name is applied to the clinical syndrome?

(d) What is the primary disease?

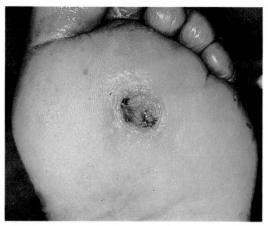

118 A 50-year-old Indian presented with a lesion on the sole of his foot.
(a) What is the lesion?
(b) Under what circumstances does it arise?
(c) Would biopsy of the lesion establish the cause?
(d) Would a serological test be helpful?
(e) Would biopsy of some other tissue give the diagnosis?

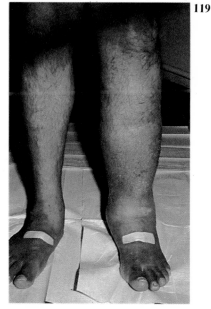

119 A 45-year-old man spent his first 20 years in India. For the past 15 years he has suffered recurrent cellulitis of one leg, with progressive swelling.
(a) What is the condition?
(b) What is the basic pathological lesion?
(c) List three causes of the condition.

120

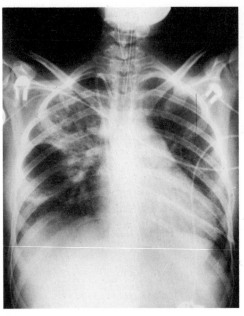

120 A girl received a bone marrow transplant for the treatment of leukaemia; 2 weeks later she became febrile and blood cultures gave a growth of *Staphylococcus aureus*. The infection responded to treatment with antibiotics and her condition improved. Nine weeks after transplant her temperature rose; she became dyspnoeic.
(a) What does the chest X-ray show?
(b) Did the staphylococcal infection involve the lungs?
(c) Would the late-stage febrile illness be caused by the infection?
(d) What are the probable causes of lung disease at this stage?

121 A 32-year-old woman had been in East Africa for the previous 8 weeks. Three weeks ago she developed pyrexia and was given tablets for 3 days to treat malaria. She improved until 2 days ago. Today, on returning to a temperate climate, her temperature is 38.5°C.
(a) What does the blood film show?
(b) Does she need treatment?
(c) Was her illness 3 weeks ago due to malaria?
(d) Is she infectious to a biting mosquito?
(e) Is she now immune to malaria?

121

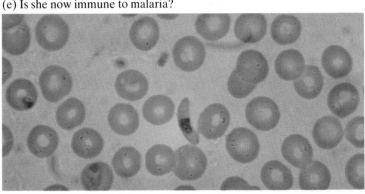

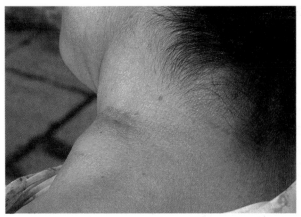

122 An Indian woman presented with a swelling in the neck, which had been present for several weeks and had increased in size. There was very little constitutional upset.

a) Is a non-infective cause more probable than an infective one?
b) Is it likely that similar swellings are present at other sites?
c) Will the chest X-ray be abnormal?
d) Will an immunological test be of value?
e) How will the diagnosis be confirmed?

123 A 30-year-old man had recurrent attacks of urethritis, arthritis and conjunctivitis. He had a rash on the soles of his feet and lesions on his glans penis.
(a) What is the probable diagnosis?
(b) What is the term applied to the rash?
(c) What is the aetiology?
(d) What late complication may develop in the eye?

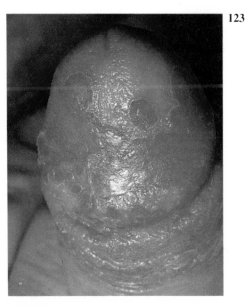

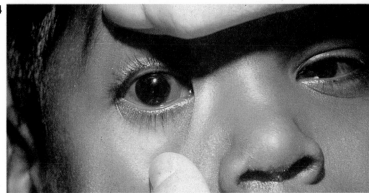

124 A young boy had a troublesome cough associated with vomiting. After a bout of coughing he developed a very red eye.
(a) What is the nature of the eye lesion?
(b) What is the probable cause of his cough?
(c) How would the diagnosis be confirmed?
(d) What is the prognosis for the eye condition?

125 A 32-year-old man living in the Sudan developed mild left-sided chest pain six months ago. Chest X-ray showed a single well-circumscribed homogeneous opacity about 4 cm in diameter at the left base. Today he had a sudden bout of coughing and produced about 50 ml of thin watery sputum.
(a) What does the sputum microscopy show?
(b) What is the relationship between the sputum findings and the clinical and radiological features?
(c) Are any other investigations indicated?
(d) Following the bout of coughing, would you expect other clinical features to appear?

125

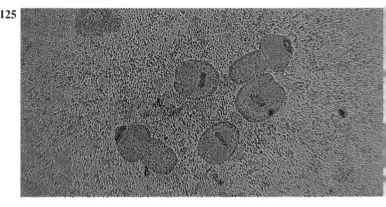

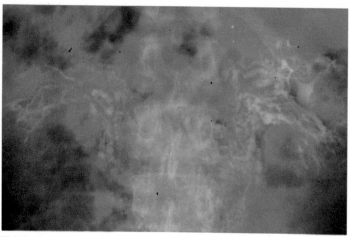

126 This is the bilateral lymphangiogram of an Indian patient with urinary symtoms.
(a) Is there an abnormality of the X-ray?
(b) What does the patient complain of?
(c) What is the most probable diagnosis?

127 A week-old-baby became ill and was thought to have neonatal sepsis. The initial manifestation was conjunctivitis, followed by lethargy and failure to thrive. After a series of convulsions he became comatosed and had an ocular palsy. He died without regaining conciousness. At autopsy foci of miliary necrosis were found in many organs.
(a) What abnormality is present in this section of liver?
(b) What infection caused death?
(c) What is the source of the infection?
(d) What are the risks of neonatal infection when the mother is infected?

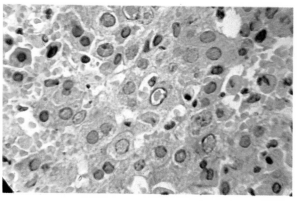

128

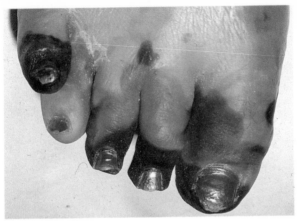

128 During the course of a severe feverish illness a boy's toes altered in appearance and became cold to the touch.
(a) What was the nature of the illness?
(b) What is the complication?
(c) What organisms probably caused the illness?
(d) Would there be any disorder of blood clotting?

129 This patient had been on safari in Zimbabwe and developed a high fever. He had many small skin lesions, thought to be insect bites.
(a) Is the appearance of this blood film related to his febrile illness?
(b) Are other investigations needed before reaching a diagnosis?
(c) Are other investigations needed before starting treatment?
(d) If he is not treated will other abnormal physical signs appear?
(e) What is the prognosis if he is not treated?

129

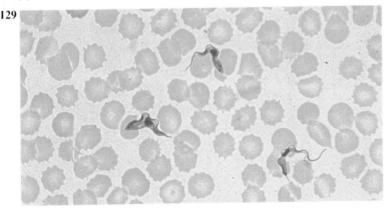

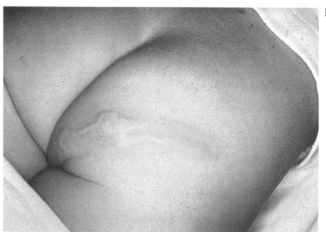

130 A man developed a rash on his buttock. He had felt unwell for some months with flatulent dyspepsia and intermittent mild diarrhoea, accompanied by some loss of weight. A blood count showed a marked eosinophilia.
(a) What is the cause of the skin lesion?
(b) Which agent is probably responsible?
(c) How would the diagnosis be confirmed?
(d) Is this condition important in the immunocompromised patient?

131 (a) What abnormalities are present in this section of skin?
(b) What is the differential diagnosis?
(c) What infective agents may be responsible?

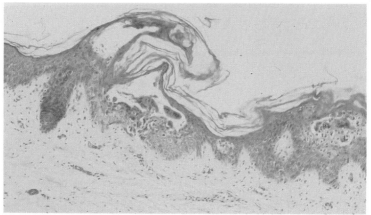

132

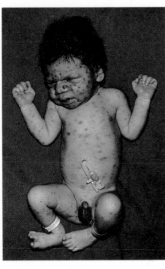

132 A baby, born in England, was found to have a haemorrhagic rash at delivery.
(a) What is the most probable diagnosis?
(b) How would the diagnosis be confirmed?
(c) At what stage of pregnancy is the infection most likely to have occurred?
(d) What other defects may be present?
(e) What is the prognosis?

133 This is a biopsy from a 40-year-old East African woman, who had an abnormality in her stool.
(a) What is the tissue biopsied?
(b) What is the abnormality?
(c) What is the cause of the abnormality?
(d) What was found on stool examination?
(e) Is treatment indicated?

133

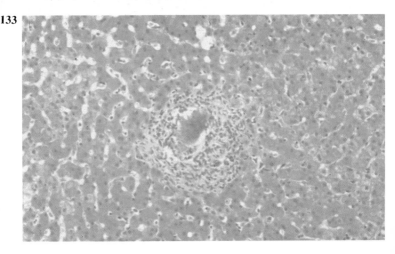

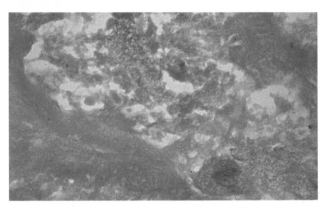

134 A 30-year-old man from North Africa was admitted with a 4-week history of low fever and some shortness of breath. He had an aortic diastolic murmur. Chest X-ray showed cardiac enlargement. Repeated blood cultures were sterile. His condition deteriorated with signs of congestive heart failure, so his aortic valve was replaced. A photomicrograph of the valve section is shown. Five years previously he had been told that he had a heart murmur.

(a) What is the sequence of events in this patient?
(b) What is the aetiology?
(c) What is the cause of the previously noted cardiac murmur?
(d) How was the aetiological diagnosis made?
(e) How is the condition acquired?

135 (a) What lesion is shown?
(b) What organism is responsible?
(c) What other site is likely to be colonised by the organism?
(d) What is the epidemiology of recurring lesions of this type?

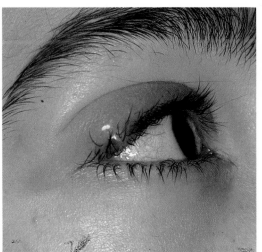

136

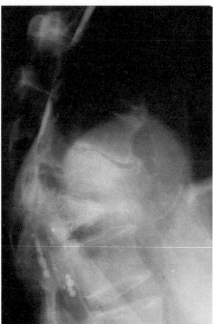

136 A man aged 40 years, who has lived mainly in Cyprus, has suffered for 2 months from pain in his back. There is a mild deformity in the lumbar region.
(a) What are the radiological abnormalities?
(b) What is the differential diagnosis?
(c) Is he likely to have other symptoms?
(d) How could the diagnosis be confirmed?

137 A boy developed bilateral swelling of his face.
(a) What is the most probable diagnosis?
(b) What organism is responsible?
(c) For how long will he remain infectious?
(d) Would the serum amylase be increased?

137

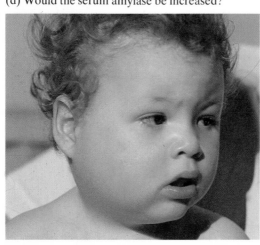

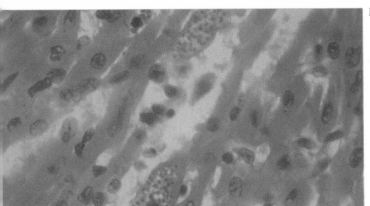

138 A 10-year-old Brazilian girl felt unwell, with fever and swelling of her left eye. Over 2 weeks she developed non-tender swelling of the axillary and inguinal lymph nodes, and some oedema of her feet. Tachycardia and an irregular pulse were noted 4 weeks ago. Cardiac failure led to death.
(a) What does the section of heart muscle show?
(b) Is death the usual outcome of this disorder?
(c) If she had survived, how could the diagnosis have been made?
(d) If she had survived the acute phase, what would the course of her illness have been?

139 A teenager developed a solitary scaly macule on his neck. A week later a generalised rash appeared, consisting of smaller oval macules, heaviest on the trunk and proximal parts of the limbs.
a) What is the probable diagnosis?
b) What other signs may be present?
c) For how long will the rash persist?
d) How infectious is the disease?

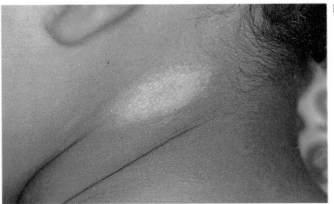

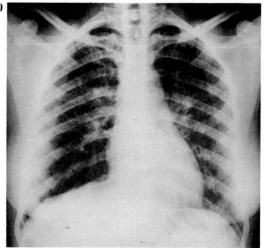

140 A 26-year-old West African woman presented with a 4 week history of pain in her chest and some arthralgia. A tuberculin test with 5 TU was positive, with induration of 10 mm in diameter after 48 hours. The absolute eosinophil count was 0.8 X 10^9/l. The toxoplasma dye test was positive at 1 : 8000. Hookworm ova were present in her stool.
(a) What does the chest radiograph show?
(b) What is the differential diagnosis based on the X-ray appearance?
(c) What is the diagnosis?
(d) What is the prognosis?
(e) Should any advice be given to the patient?

141 (a) What deformities are present?
(b) What are the probable causes?
(c) How would the diagnosis be established?

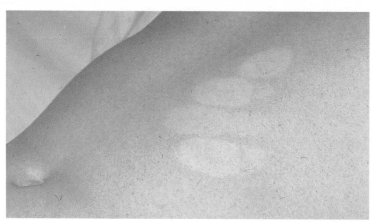

142 A young woman suddenly became ill with a high fever, conjunctivitis, an erythematous rash, diarrhoea and circulatory collapse. There was marked myalgia, and the blood level of creatinine phosphokinase was strikingly elevated.
(a) What is the name of the syndrome?
(b) Where is the common site of the infection?
(c) What organism is responsible?

143 A girl developed a fever and flu-like symptoms. Next day a rash appeared. Her throat was inflamed but there were no other respiratory symptoms or signs. The illness settled after 5 days.
(a) What is the differential diagnosis?
(b) What is the probable causative agent?
(c) Where would it be detected?
(d) What other syndromes may be associated with this agent?

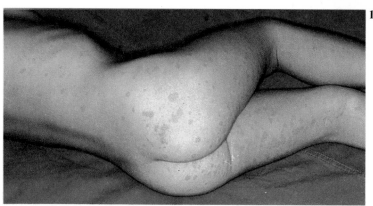

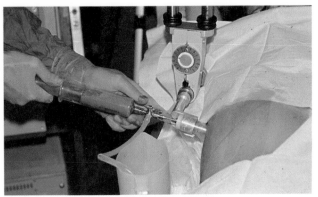

144 A 35-year-old man had been in West Africa for 2 years. During the previous 3 weeks he had been unwell with pyrexia, loss of weight and pain in his right lower chest. His white blood cell count was 16×10^9/l.
(a) What procedure is being carried out?
(b) Under what circumstances is it indicated?
(c) What would a chest X-ray show?
(d) What other investigations would be helpful?
(e) What is the diagnosis?

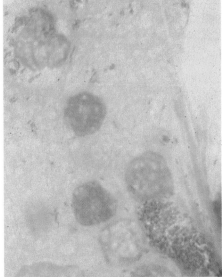

145 A 17-year-old Indian boy lives in India. Four weeks ago, a lump appeared on the right side of his neck, increasing to 2 cm diameter. No other swellings. He is a febrile and feels fairly well.
(a) What does the biospy of the mass show?
(b) Is the tuberculin test of such value in this situation that biopsy is unnecessary?
(c) What would a chest X-ray be expected to show?
(d) How did he become infected?
(e) Should he be isolated?

146 A Sudanese woman presented with multiple lesions on her lower thigh, which had been present for 9 months. There were black granules in the discharge from the lesions. The limb was not very painful; little constitutional upset; physical examination otherwise normal.

(a) What differential diagnosis is suggested by the X-ray?

(b) Would examination of the discharge be helpful?

(c) What is the most probable diagnosis and how may it be established?

(d) Is local or metastatic spread likely?

(e) How is the condition acquired?

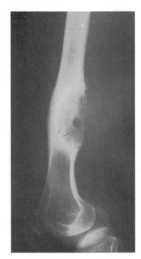

146

147 An African boy had a skin lesion, quickly followed by multiple similar lesions, which had been present for about 3 weeks. They were not painful or very itchy. Little constitutional upset.

(a) What is the diagnosis?

(b) What is the natural evolution of these superficial skin lesions?

(c) May there be involvement of bones?

(d) May there be visceral involvement?

(e) How may the diagnosis be confirmed?

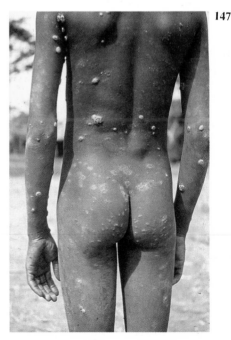

147

148

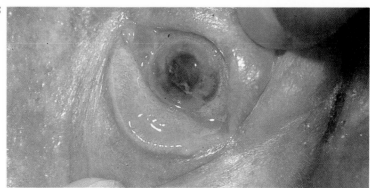

148 Following an attack of herpes zoster involving the ophthalmic division of the fifth cranial nerve, this patient had a red watering eye.
(a) What abnormality is present?
(b) What is the cause of this condition?
(c) What complications may develop?
(d) What treatment is required?

149 A 22-year-old man from West Africa was killed in a road accident 4 days previously.
(a) What does the spleen show?
(b) What is the probable source of the abnormality?
(c) Is the finding likely to have been associated with ill-health in the past?
(d) Is the finding itself of importance?
(e) Could it have been prevented?

149

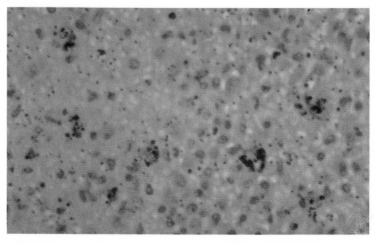

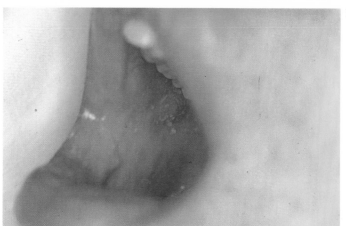

150 A boy developed a fever with acute respiratory symptoms. After 2 days he complained of abdominal pain and began to vomit.
(a) What can be seen in his mouth?
(b) What is the diagnosis?
(c) What is the probable cause of his abdominal pain?
(d) Should he be treated conservatively?

151 A 30-year-old woman spent 3 weeks in South Africa and visited game parks. A few days after leaving Africa she developed a lesion on her buttock only, which increased to its present size over 7 days. She felt mildly unwell but no marked constitutional upset.
(a) Is this skin lesion especially related to her visit to South Africa?
(b) How did the lesion arise?
(c) What is the differential diagnosis?
(d) How is the diagnosis made with certainty?
(e) What will happen to the lesion?

151

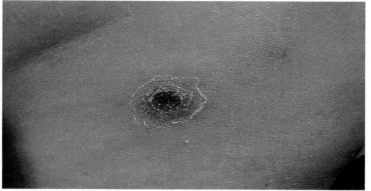

152 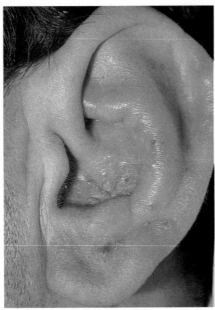 During the course of a severe attack of pneumococcal meningitis this man developed a rash on his pinna.

(a) What is the nature of the rash?

(b) What is the causative organism?

(c) What is the relationship between this condition and the attack of meningitis?

(d) Are serological tests helpful in diagnosing this condition?

153 A man spent 4 years in India until 12 years ago. He has suffered symptoms intermittently over the past 2 years.

(a) What is the condition of his left leg?

(b) What other symptoms is he likely to have?

(c) What is the differential diagnosis?

(d) Are there any long-term sequelae?

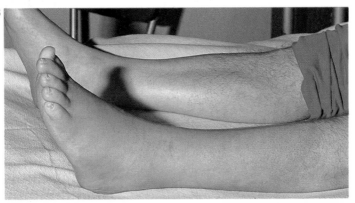

154 A man was admitted to hospital with a 1 day history of stiffness of his neck and difficulty in walking. He had difficulty in swallowing and showed this appearance.

(a) What is this facial expression called?

(b) What is the underlying condition?

(c) How is the condition acquired?

(d) Do any factors influence the prognosis?

(e) Can treatment influence the outcome?

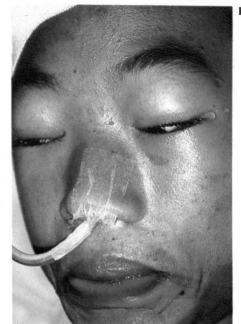

154

155 A 40-year-old man presented a 6-month history of irritating cough and hoarse voice.

(a) What does the radiograph show?

(b) What might be heard on auscultation?

(c) What is the aetiology?

(d) What is the pathogenesis?

(e) What is the prognosis?

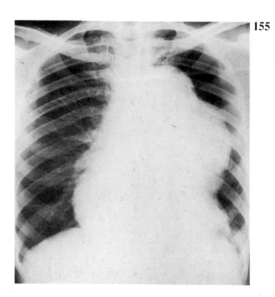

155

156

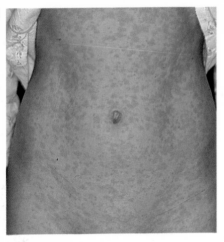

156 A young girl developed fever, coryza and a troublesome dry cough. She was treated with an antibiotic for a respiratory tract infection. After 4 days a rash appeared behind her ears and on the back of her neck which spread downwards over the next 2 days to cover her whole body.

(a) What is the diagnosis?

(b) Is the treatment the cause of her rash?

(c) What other signs would be present?

(d) What complications may develop?

157 A 26-year-old man worked in a refugee camp in Africa for 9 months. Two days ago he developed fever and headache. A lumbar puncture was carried out today.

(a) What does the Gram stain of the CSF show?

(b) What would be the expected CSF cell count?

(c) What would be the expected CSF protein and sugar?

(d) Would this patient have a positive blood culture?

(e) Would skin lesions be found?

157

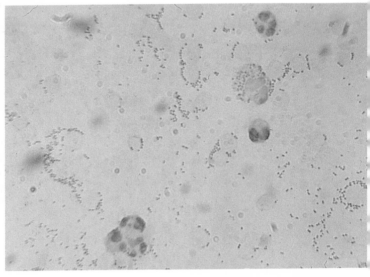

158 A 52-year-old Egyptian presented with a 6-month history of general ill-health and loss of weight; 1 month ago he had noticed swelling of his abdomen. His liver was greatly enlarged and hard but only slightly tender. His mucosae were pale but he was not jaundiced.
(a) What is the differential diagnosis?
(b) How may the diagnosis be established?
(c) What is the role of infection in this disorder?
(d) Could this disorder have been prevented?
(e) What is the prognosis?

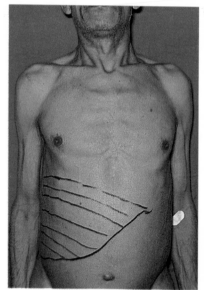

158

159 A 35-year-old man left India 5 years ago to live in a temperate climate. Three years ago he noticed swelling of his foot, together with a number of skin lesions, which discharged intermittently. His skin was clear elsewhere and there was no constitutional upset.
(a) What sort of organism is responsible for this infection?
(b) What is the mode of transmission?
(c) How may the diagnosis be made?
(d) Is spread from this site likely?
(e) What would an X-ray of the foot show?

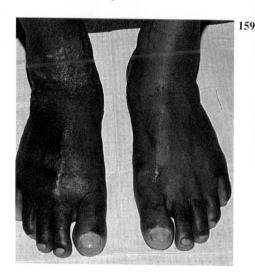

159

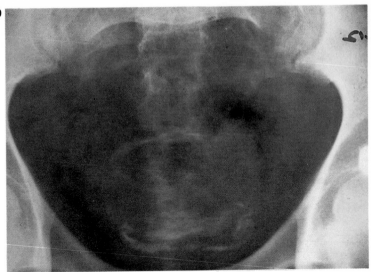

160 A 30-year-old Egyptian received treatment for haematuria at 12 years-of-age. There has been no recurrence of bleeding.
(a) What is the radiological abnormality?
(b) What is the pathological change underlying the radiological abnormality?
(c) What is the differential diagnosis?
(d) Are there any local or distal complications of this condition?

161 (a) What is the nature of the lesion of this child's eye?
(b) What is the prognosis?

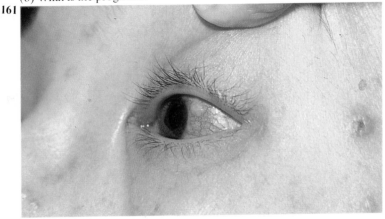

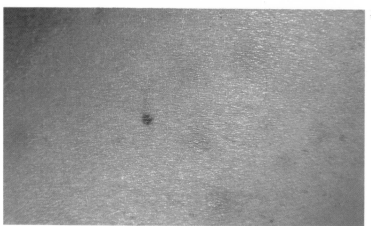

162 A man went on safari to a game reserve in East Africa. A week later he became ill with a fever, severe headache and myalgia. After 4 days an erythematous macular rash appeared, heaviest over the trunk and lower limbs.
(a) Would any other signs be expected?
(b) What is the diagnosis?
(c) What is the causative organism?
(d) Would the rash become haemorrhagic?
(e) What is the prognosis?

163 An elderly woman was admitted to hospital with a painful rash.
(a) What has caused the rash?
(b) What other abnormalities are present?
(c) What is the underlying pathology?

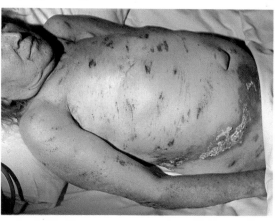

164

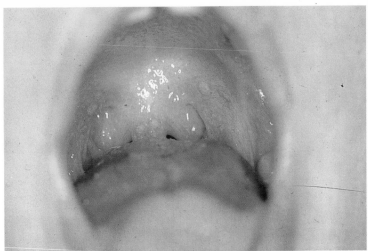

164 A girl became ill with a fever, sore throat and dysphagia, and complained of headache, myalgia and pain in her abdomen.
(a) What is the diagnosis?
(b) What is the cause?
(c) What is the course of the illness?

165 A 24-year-old man lived in Cameroun, West Africa. He is troubled by skin irritation for which he was given tablets several years ago. There is a maculo-papular rash on his shoulders and buttocks.
(a) What does the skin snip of an infected area show?
(b) Why should his eyes be examined?
(c) What may happen following the start of treatment?
(d) Is treatment likely to cure his symptoms?
(e) Could the condition have been prevented?

165

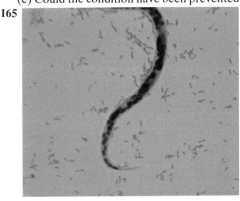

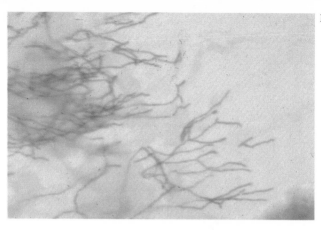

166 A 40-year-old man noticed a painless swelling under his chin 4 months ago. It enlarged and has discharged from more than one site. The mass was indurated and discharging thin purulent material, in which was seen a yellow particle. This was crushed and stained. His teeth were in poor condition.
(a) What does the stained material show?
(b) What is the nature of the infecting organism?
(c) What is the nature of the yellow particle?
(d) How was the infection acquired?
(e) What is the prognosis?

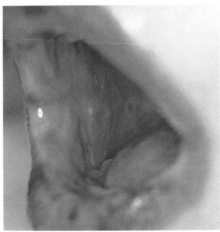

167 A woman became ill with a high fever, an extensive pleomorphic painless rash, sore eyes, a painful mouth and dysuria.
(a) What is the diagnosis?
(b) What is the cause of the condition?
(c) What is the usual course of the illness?
(d) What other structures may be involved in addition to the skin and mucous membranes?

168 A girl in Thailand suddenly developed a high fever and non-specific symptoms. It persisted for 4 days, then subsided. As her temperature dropped a petechial rash appeared. At this stage her platelet count was found to be low.
(a) What is the most probable diagnosis?
(b) What is the infecting agent?
(c) How is it spread?
(d) What serious complication may develop?

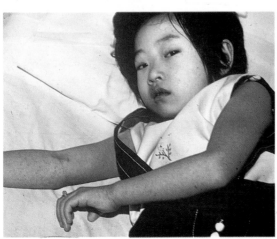

169 A man became ill with a sore throat. He was afebrile and there was very little disturbance. He had marked halitosis.
(a) What is the diagnosis?
(b) What is the cause?
(c) What are the predisposing factors?

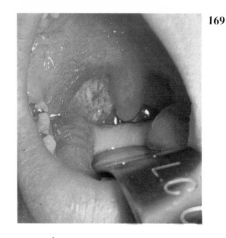

170 A young man was treated for an attack of meningitis accompanied by a generalised petechial rash. During convalescence he complained of painful swelling of his knees.
(a) What type of meningitis did he have?
(b) What is the cause of his painful knees?
(c) What would aspiration of the knee joint reveal?
(d) What is the prognosis?

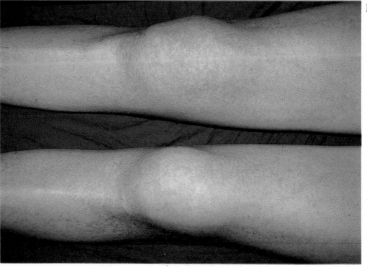

171

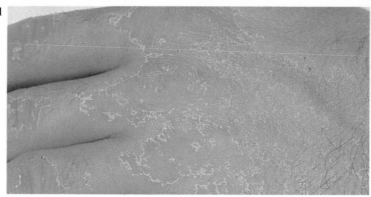

171 (a) What condition is shown?
(b) Is it characteristic of scarlet fever?
(c) Where does this condition begin in scarlet fever?
(d) Are the squames infectious in scarlet fever?

172 A Sikh aged 27 years came to Britain from India last year. Six weeks ago he developed intermittent pyrexia and felt generally unwell. He was febrile, there were two lymph nodes palpable in his neck and the tip of his spleen could be felt. His white blood cell count was 5.6×10^9/l and his ESR 30 mm in 1 hour.
(a) What is the differential diagnosis?
(b) Would a skin test be of value?
(c) Would a sputum examination be helpful?
(d) Would a bone marrow aspirate give the diagnosis?
(e) What procedure would be most likely to provide the diagnosis?

172

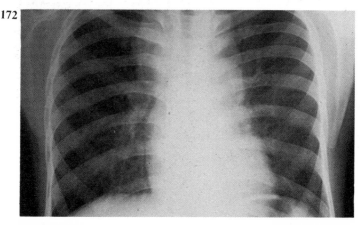

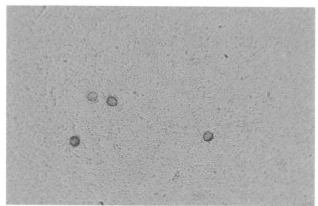

173 A 6-year-old boy presented with a 24-hour history of increasing watery diarrhoea and is now passing stools every hour. He has vomited twice and complains of abdominal pain. No previous illnesses; his family is not affected.
(a) What does stool microscopy show?
(b) What staining methods are suitable for demonstrating this organism?
(c) What is the probable source of the infection?

174 A 33-year-old man had been in Egypt for some years. He presented with pain in his neck, low pyrexia and general ill-health.
(a) What abnormality does this X-ray of his spine show?
(b) What is the differential diagnosis?
(c) Is he likely to have other bony lesions?
(d) If the underlying cause is removed will the radiological changes disappear?
(e) How would the diagnosis be made?

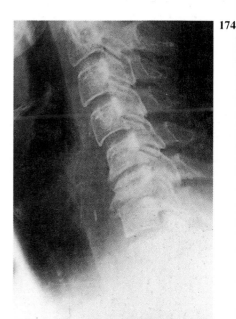

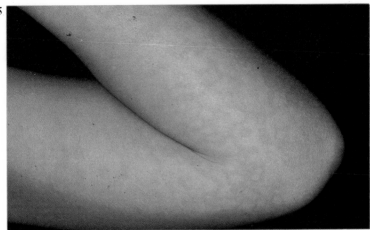

175 A boy presented with a fever, tachycardia, joint pains and an extensive rash.
(a) What is the nature of the rash?
(b) What is the diagnosis?
(c) How would the diagnosis be confirmed?
(d) Is he infectious?

176 A patient complained of pain in left side of his face and palate for three days before an eruption appeared.
(a) What is the probable diagnosis?
(b) Is he likely to have a rash elsewhere?
(c) How will the palatal lesions evolve?
(d) Will there be any sequelae?

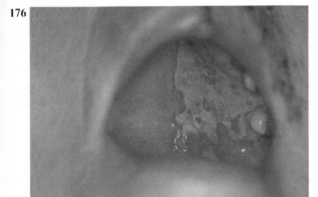

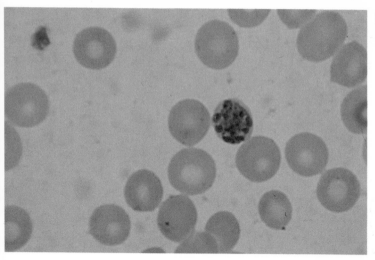

177 A 40-year-old man lived in the tropics for about 18 years, and came to Britain 6 weeks ago. Abroad, he often suffered from diarrhoea and was treated for 'malaria' on many occasions. One week ago he developed pyrexia and headache which have persisted intermittently. His spleen is easily palpable on inspiration and his haemoglobin is 11.2 g/dl.
(a) What does the peripheral blood film show?
(b) When did he develop this condition?
(c) What is the relationship between the clinical features and the blood film findings?
(d) What will be the effect of a schizontocide?
(e) Are there any complications of this condition?

178

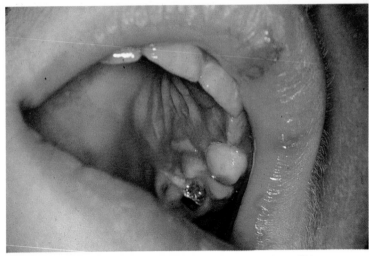

178 A man complained to his dentist of painful ulceration of his gums.
(a) What is the differential diagnosis?
(b) Is this likely to be a primary attack?
(c) How would the diagnosis be confirmed?
(d) What is the probability of recurrent attacks?

179 This chest X-ray is of a young child with a cardiac murmur.
(a) What infection probably caused the heart disease?
(b) What other defects may be present?
(c) For how long may the child remain infectious?

180 A woman developed painless swelling of her anterior cervical lymph nodes, felt unwell and had some loss of weight. Chest X-ray was normal; Mantoux test strongly positive. Lymph nodes on the right side of her neck were biopsied. Histologically there were caseating granulomas.

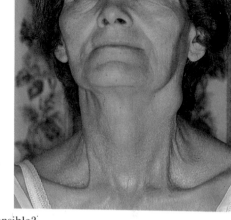

(a) What is the diagnosis?
(b) What proportion of patients with this condition would have active pulmonary involvement?
(c) What organism is responsible?
(d) What surgical complication is present?

181 A 36-year-old woman lived in Hong Kong. Three weeks ago she became ill with pyrexia which worsened and she developed rigors. Two weeks ago she became jaundiced, at which time her liver was palpable and tender. *Escherichia coli* was cultured from her blood. At operation, the bile duct was drained. Despite chemotherapy she died 3 days ago.

(a) What does the liver section show?
(b) Is the section finding related to her illness?
(c) How was the liver finding acquired?
(d) Is her illness the usual outcome of the infection shown in the section?
(e) Are there other serious consequences of the infection?

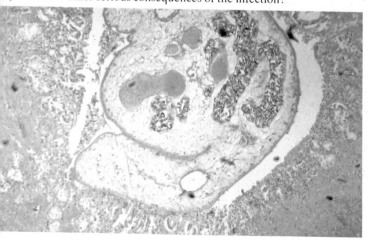

182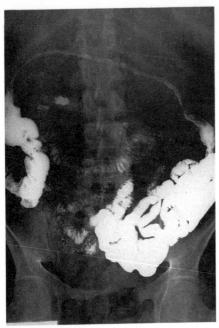

182 An Indian woman complained of abdominal pain of 6-months' duration. Examination revealed a mass in the upper quadrant. A barium enema was performed.
(a) What is the radiological abnormality?
(b) What is the most probable diagnosis?
(c) How may the diagnosis be confirmed?
(d) What did the histology of the bowel show?

183 (a) What is this condition?
(b) Which organism is responsible?
(c) What is the source of the infection?
(d) What are the predisposing causes?

183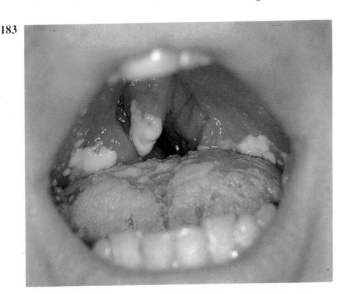

184 A patient developed a rash, consisting of small red slightly elevated papules and vesicles, unevenly distributed and intensely itchy, especially when he was warm. A close-up of one of the lesions is shown.

(a) What is the diagnosis?
(b) What is the distribution of the rash?
(c) What organism is responsible?
(d) What is the source?
(e) How is it spread?

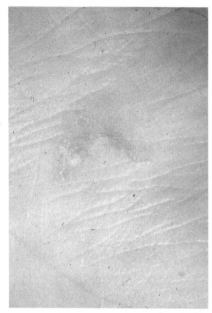

185 A young woman developed a lesion on the skin of her face in early childhood. This has progressed over many years to involve a large area of her face.

(a) What is the differential diagnosis?
(b) How may the diagnosis be confirmed?
(c) How is the infection acquired?
(d) What is the prognosis?

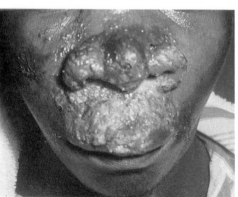

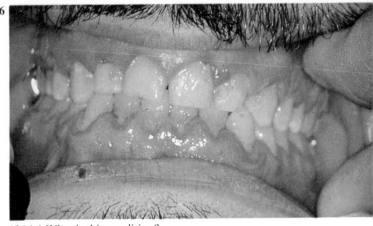

186 (a) What is this condition?
(b) What organisms are responsible?
(c) What are the predisposing causes?

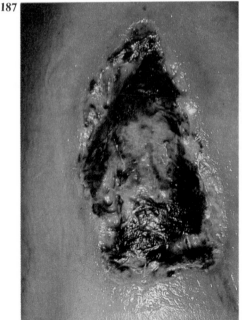

187 A middle-aged man developed a painless lump on the medial aspect of his thigh. It enlarged steadily over some weeks before the central area broke down to form a large painless ulcer. No constitutional disturbance.

(a) What is the probable diagnosis?
(b) How could the diagnosis be confirmed?
(c) What is the natural course of the illness?
(d) What is the pathological process?

188 A young child developed a painful swelling at the angle of the jaw, accompanied by feverishness and malaies.
(a) Is this mumps?
(b) What is the nature of the swelling?
(c) What organism is probably responsible?
(d) What would the white blood cell count be?

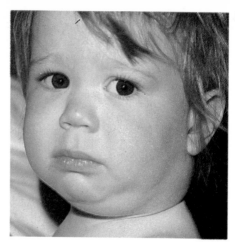

189 A man developed headache, shivering, myalgia and marked lassitude, followed by a sore throat and, later, a distressing cough producing thick mucoid sputum. No respiratory distress and few signs on clinical examination of the chest. White blood cell count was $11 \times 10^9/l$ and ESR 85 mm in the first hour. Cold agglutinins were detected in his blood.
(a) What is the probable diagnosis?
(b) What is the causative organism?
(c) What is the natural course of the illness?
(d) How could the diagnosis be confirmed?
(e) What complications may develop?

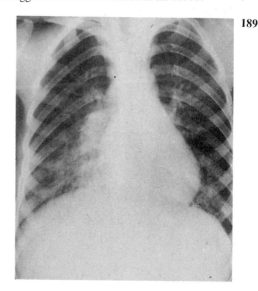

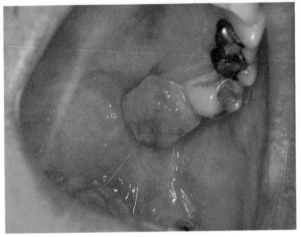

190 A 40-year-old Englishman developed a scanty rash of pigmented papules on his legs, accompanied by a small tumour in his mouth. There was generalised enlargement of his lymph nodes.
(a) What is the diagnosis?
(b) What is the underlying disease?
(c) What investigations may prove helpful?
(d) What is the prognosis?

191 A woman had a short attack of diarrhoea about 3 weeks ago. A week later she felt unwell with a low fever and puffiness of the eyes, followed by myalgia. Her absolute eosinophil count is $1.2 \times 10^9/l$ and she has a tender swelling of the left biceps which was biopsied.

191

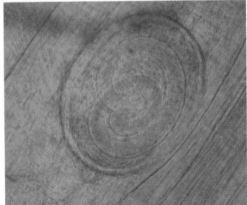

(a) What does the section show?
(b) Is the biopsy finding related to her illness?
(c) How is the infection acquired?
(d) Could the diagnosis have been made without biopsy?
(e) What is the prognosis?

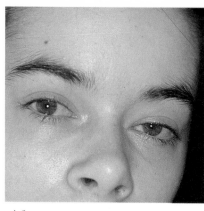

192 A month after acquiring a puppy, this woman became ill with a fever and a very severe headache. She had neck stiffness and photophobia. A lumbar puncture was performed and her CSF was found to contain 450 cells/mm^3, with a preponderance of mononuclear cells.

(a) What is the differential diagnosis?
(b) What organism is probably responsible?
(c) Would it be found in the CSF?
(d) How is the diagnosis usually confirmed?
(e) Is she likely to develop renal failure?

193 A 4-year-old Nigerian boy who lived in southern Nigeria presented 3 days ago with massive generalised oedema, which involved his scalp, making it difficult for him to open his eyes. His urine contains protein 6 g/l and his serum albumin is 8 g/l.

(a) What does the blood film show?
(b) Are the clinical features and the blood film findings related?
(c) What is the pathogenesis of this condition?
(d) What will be the effect of a schizontocide?
(e) What is the prognosis?

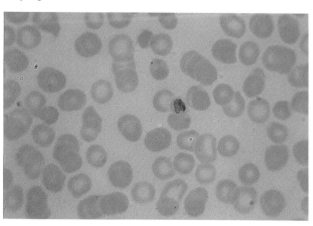

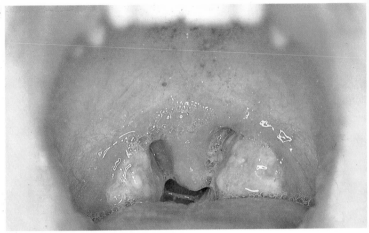

194 A young man in London became ill with a sore throat and a fever of 38.6°C.
(a) What is shown?
(b) What is the most probable diagnosis?
(c) What other physical signs may be present?
(d) How could the diagnosis be confirmed?

195 Both of these African children are 3 years old. The one on the right has had repeated respiratory infections and measles. A year ago her haemoglobin level was 8 g/dl and sickle-cell anaemia was confirmed. Two days ago the mother noticed her paleness and her haemoglobin level was found to be 3.5 g/dl with 0.1% reticulocytes.

195

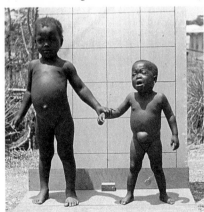

(a) What has happened?
(b) What is the significance of the reticulocyte count?
(c) What is the aetiology of the condition?
(d) Is she likely to have repeated crises?
(e) What is the management?

196 A girl developed a mild illness with a slightly sore throat. Next day an erythematous rash appeared on her face and limbs but not on her trunk, palms or soles. Over several days the rash faded and reappeared, finally disappearing after 5 days.

(a) What is the diagnosis?
(b) What is the cause?
(c) Does the condition occur in adults?
(d) What is the prognosis?

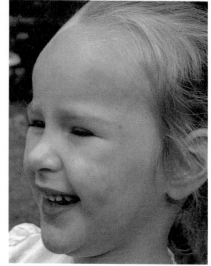

197 A young woman developed a feverish illness with painful swelling of her knee, elbow and wrist joints. She had a sparse rash on the distal parts of her limbs, consisting of small haemorrhagic pustules on an erythematous base.

(a) What is the differential diagnosis?
(b) How would the diagnosis be confirmed?
(c) Where is the primary site of infection?
(d) Would it be clinically evident?
(e) What complications may develop?

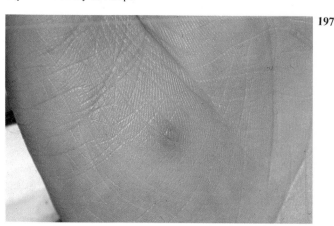

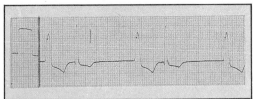

198 A previously healthy child was admitted to hospital 10 days after the onset of illness.
(a) What does the ECG show?
(b) What is the probable cause?
(c) What other system may be affected and when?
(d) What is the prognosis?

199 A young girl presented with tender swelling of her supra- and infraclavicular lymph nodes. The epitrochlear node was enlarged but not tender. The nodes were not fluctuant and there was no lymphangitis. She felt mildly unwell and denied having had any lesion on her hand or forearm. She lived in England and had never been abroad. A month previously she had looked after a cat.
(a) What is the diagnosis?
(b) How could the diagnosis be confirmed?
(c) What is the prognosis?

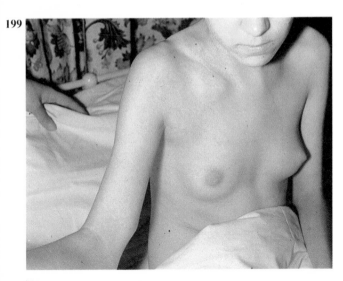

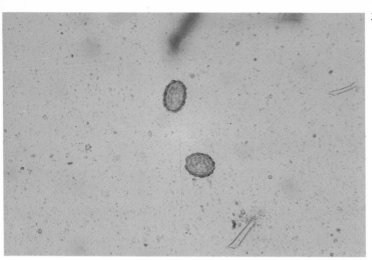

200 A 24-year-old man has been in India for 6-months. Recently he suffered many attacks of diarrhoea which have now become continuous. He has a lot of flatulence and abdominal distension. His appetite and energy are poor and he has lost 9 kg in weight.
(a) What does stool microscopy show?
(b) What is the relationship between the stool findings and his symptoms?
(c) Are futher investigations indicated?
(d) What would jejunal aspirate show?
(e) What is the probable diagnosis?

ANSWERS

1 (a) Herpes simplex.

(b) Yes. In a child it may be a component of a primary infection involving the mouth.

(c) It would be most unusual.

(d) Doctors and nurses are especially prone to herpetic lesions on fingers as a result of exposure to infected secretions from patients.

2 (a) Diffuse fine nodular shadowing in the right lung.

(b) Exposure to birds and the clinical combination of pneumonitis with splenomegaly point to a diagnosis of ornithosis.

(c) *Chlamydia psittaci*, an obligate intracellular parasite possessing both DNA and RNA.

(d) By demonstrating a rising antibody level in paired sera.

(e) *Chlamydia psittaci* has been demonstrated in nearly 100 species of birds. Man can be infected by inhaling dust from dried faeces or feathers, or by handling carcasses of infected birds, such as ducks or turkeys.

3 (a) This rests between Stevens–Johnson syndrome and acute toxic epidermal necrolysis (scalded-skin syndrome). The painful skin and the separation of the epidermis from the underlying layers point to the latter.

(b) Usually caused by an exotoxin produced by *Staphylococcus aureus* belonging to phage group II. Staphylococcus may be present on the skin but is more frequently found at another site.

(c) Nikolsky's sign.

(d) The skin lesions heal in about 2 weeks, usually without scarring.

4 (a) Trophozoites of *Giardia lamblia*.

(b) *Gardia lamblia* is a cause of diarrhoea, and the presence of trophozoites rather than cysts favours the parasite as the cause.

(c) Giardiasis may give rise to malabsorption and weight loss is a feature. If this were investigated, then urinary xylose excretion, faecal fat and the Schilling test would be appropriate.

(d) Although the parasite may be eradicated by treatment, some patients continue to pass loose stools for some time. Lactase deficiency may persist after tests of absorption have returned to normal.

(e) By ingestion of cysts, usually from water.

5 (a) Enlarged hilar lymph nodes.

(b) Tuberculosis.

(c) This is a primary infection with the tubercle bacillus, where the organism has lodged in the periphery of the lung, producing a Ghon focus. Subsequent lymphatic spread to the hilar lymph nodes results in a primary complex. In most cases the primary complex heals uneventfully but it may proceed to caseation or post-primary infection. In young children, the lung component may be too small to see; the main feature is the glandular involvement.

(d) By development of tuberculin sensitivity or the detection of tubercle bacilli in gastric washings. Laboratory confirmation is rarely obtained.

6 (a) Trophozoites (rings) of *Plasmodium falciparum*. Some red cells contain more than one parasite and some cells show accolé forms, where the parasite lies against the cell membrane. About 25 per cent of the cells are parasitised; this is a heavy infection.

(b) Abnormal behaviour is not uncommon in malignant tertian malaria. It is thought that its basis is similar to that of the other manifestations of complicated malaria, namely occlusion of small blood vessels by red cells contain-

ing dividing parasites (schizogony).
(c) This is a medical emergency; immediate parenteral treatment should result in a 90 per cent recovery rate.
(d) Parasites will continue to be seen within red cells in reduced numbers but do not undergo division. In some patients gametocytes (sexual forms) appear after recovery.

7 (a) This rests between contagious pustular dermatitis (orf) and paravaccina (milkers' nodes). The papule of orf develops into a large flat vesicle or bulla, which may be haemorrhagic, whereas the lesion of paravaccinia does not. Orf is derived from sheep or goats, paravaccinia from cattle.
(b) Paravaccinia virus, a double-stranded DNA virus belonging to the *Poxviridae*.
(c) Severe allergic rashes.
(d) No.

8 (a) The conjunctiva is injected and there are haemorrhages.
(b) She has a purpuric rash.
(c) It is likely to be meningococcal.
(d) Disseminated intravascular coagulation and, possibly, Waterhouse-Friderichsen syndrome.
(e) A low platelet count, prolonged prothrombin and thrombin times, low fibrinogen and high fibrin degradation product levels.

9 (a) Marked changes—especially in the metatarsals, where there is erosion and destruction of bone.
(b) The hand-foot syndrome, which here involves the feet only, is not uncommon in small children, homozygous for the sickle-cell gene. This baby had sickle-cell anaemia.
(c) Yes. The changes could be the result of osteomyelitis; in fact *Haemophilus influenzae* was grown from the blood.
(d) These are common in sickle-cell anaemia and are of two main types: those due to an expanded bone marrow and those due to infarction.
(e) No. There is a high mortality among young children with sickle-cell disease, due mainly to infection, to which they are unduly susceptible.

10 (a) Yes. The throat is usually inflamed and there may be vesicles on the tongue, palate or pharynx. It is not unusual to detect petechiae on the palate.
(b) The patient begins to shed virus a few hours before the onset of illness and remains infectious until the lesions have crusted.
(c) Vesicles form in the epidermis as a result of cellular degeneration accompanied by intracellular oedema. At first the fluid collects in small pockets which eventually merge to produce the mature vesicle. Multinucleated giant cells are formed.
(d) Secondary bacterial infection with streptococci and staphylococci.

11 (a) Tightly coiled spirochaetes about 10 μm long.
(b) Yes. The spirochaetes are *Treponema pallidum*, not commensals.
(c) Unlikely. Chloroquine seldom produces a rash and rarely caused jaundice.
(d) Pyrexia, skin rash, hepatitis with a high alkaline phosphatase level and mouth ulcers are all features of secondary syphilis, treatment for which is highly effective.

12 (a) Causes of massive splenomegaly, as illustrated, include myeloid leukaemia, myelofibrosis and visceral leishmaniasis.
(b) Bone marrow aspiration.
(c) In visceral leishmaniasis there tends to be pancytopenia.
(d) Bone marrow examination usually reveals amastigotes of *Leishmania*

donovani within macrophages. In some areas, including the Sudan, gland aspirate may show the parasite; splenic aspiration is often considered best.

13 (a) Rupture of a hydatid cyst of the lung.
(b) To remove a hydatid cyst of the liver.
(c) Scanning of the liver.
(d) No. Liver and lung are the commonest sites for hydatid cyst; she should remain under surveillance.

14 (a) An egg of *Schistosoma haematobium*; the spine is terminal.
(b) In water, schistosomal eggs hatch to release miracidia, which infect freshwater snails. After development, cercariae penetrate man's skin, resulting in adult flukes, which inhabit the venous plexus around the urinary tract. Eggs are laid there, escaping from the vessel into the lumen of the urinary tract.
(c) As the eggs leave the veins and penetrate the bladder mucosa, a small amount of blood also escapes.
(d) Intravenous pyelography and cystoscopy would enable an assessment of the degree of structural change to be made.
(e) Fibrosis in egg granulomata produces an obstructive uropathy with hydronephrosis and reduced renal function. There is also an association with squamous carcinoma of the bladder.

15 (a) Yes; small vesicles on the hands and feet.
(b) Hand, foot and mouth disease.
(c) The infection is caused by Coxsackie viruses types A16, A10 and A5.
(d) A maculo-papular rash may be present on the buttocks and the rash on the feet may be absent.

16 (a) Erysipelas.
(b) *Streptococcus pyogenes*.
(c) No, two or more attacks are quite common.
(d) The face and legs.

17 (a) Syphilis, chancroid, lymphogranuloma venereum, granuloma inguinale and herpes should be considered. The induration, lack of pain and tenderness of the lesion and inguinal gland favour a syphilitic chancre.
(b) By finding the characteristic *Treponema pallidum* on dark-field examination of the serous transudate from the ulcer. If antiseptics have been applied to the sore, repeated examinations may be necessary.
(c) The ulcer will heal over a period of weeks, perhaps leaving a small scar; the swelling of the inguinal gland may take longer to subside.
(d) A patient with untreated primary syphilis is unlikely to develop a further primary lesion if exposed.
(e) 30 per cent of patients with untreated primary syphilis used to progress to cardiovascular or neurosyphilis. These are now rare, possibly due to use of antibiotics.

18 (a) A trypanosome; the South American *Trypanosoma cruzi*.
(b) Yes, acute Chagas' disease may be present, with a lesion at the site of entry of the parasite, often the conjunctiva. The clinical features include fever and evidence of myocarditis, conduction defects or heart failure, or of encephalitis.
(c) The mortality of untreated cases is about 10 per cent.
(d) Long-term effects, such as dilatation of the heart or gut (especially of the oesophagus or colon) usually occur in patients with no history of an acute illness as in this case.
(e) Yes; infection is through faeces of reduviid bugs, which live in the walls of poorly constructed houses. The sound construction of homes virtually eliminates infection.

19 (a) Aneurysmal dilatation.

(b) Coronary artery aneurysm is an important complication of Kawasaki disease.

(c) Fever, stomatitis and pharyngitis, conjunctivitis, reddening of palms and soles, followed by membranous desquamation, exanthem and non-suppurative lymphadenopathy. Five of the six criteria must be met.

(d) Coronary thrombosis and myocardial infarction.

20 (a) A cluster of gallstones.

(b) Gallstones may be the focus of infection in a typhoid carrier.

(c) Cholecystectomy may produce a cure in 70 per cent of chronic carriers with cholelithiasis.

(d) No—the organism may be cultured from the interior of stones removed at operation.

21 (a) *Candida albicans*. This yeast infection is suggested by the well-defined area of inflammation with raised edges. Satellite lesions may begin as small pustules, which rupture to leave small areas of redness. In an ammoniacal rash, the skin folds tend to be spared.

(b) It is likely that the infection was derived from the bowel, where the yeast may have been present for some time as a commensal.

(c) The yeast tends to become pathogenic when the perineal skin becomes excessively moist as the result of diarrhoea. The use of antibiotics for the treatment of the gastro-enteritis would aggravate the situation.

22 (a) Hydrophobia.

(b) Drinking, or even the offer of a drink, puts the patient into a state of terror; there is contraction of all muscles of respiration and swallowing.

(c) Rabies.

(d) Hopeless; rabies carries virtually 100 per cent mortality.

(e) Yes. Dog bite is the commonest mode of transmission to man. If rabies vaccine had been given shortly after wounding the disease could have been prevented. Once symptoms have developed treatment has no effect.

23 (a) Cavity of the right lung, containing a fungal ball or aspergilloma.

(b) No.

(c) Colonisation of a tuberculous cavity by *Aspergillus*, most commonly *A. fumigatus*.

(d) Hyphae may be demonstrated intermittently by sputum smear, but should be confirmed by culture. IgG antibody to *Aspergillus* can be detected readily.

24 (a) Jejunum. The biopsy has been taken as part of the investigation of malabsorption.

(b) Short and blunted villi, deep crypts and a cellular infiltrate of the lamina propria.

(c) Tests of absorption, especially urinary xylose, faecal fat and vitamin B_{12} absorption (Schilling test).

(d) Barium meal and follow through would show dilatation of loops of small bowel.

(e) *Giardia lamblia*, which can be associated with malabsorption indistinguishable from tropical sprue.

25 (a) The EEG shows a striking slow wave pattern consistent with a diffuse encephalitis.

(b) Post-measles encephalitis. The essential lesion is demyelination, accompanied by microglial proliferation, possibly the result of damage from an immunological reaction.

(c) In a mild case with drowsiness and no focal signs recovery is usually complete.

26 (a) A cyst of *Entamoeba coli* stained with iodine. Note the eight nuclei.

(b) None. *Entamoeba coli* is a non-pathogenic protozoon.

(c) Yes, to discover the cause of her diarrhoea. Further stool microscopy might demonstrate *Giardia lamblia* or *Entamoeba histolytica*, and duodenal aspirate might also show *G. lamblia*. Stool culture might reveal a bacterial cause.

(d) Yes. *Entamoeba coli* is passed from man to man, usually in water.

(e) Not in that part of the bowel inspected by sigmoidoscopy. It is possible but unlikely that the colon beyond the sigmoidoscope might be affected and that *E. histolytica* may be found in a further stool specimen.

27 (a) Molluscum contagiosum.

(b) On electron microscopy inclusion bodies can be seen. These contain virions resembling poxviruses. However, a virus has not been serially propagated in tissue culture.

(c) It is long, and may extend to 50 days.

(d) By close body contact.

28 (a) Gross deformity of both lower legs, with bowing of the tibiae and marked scarring and deformity of the ankles and feet.

(b) This is tertiary yaws. Yaws is a spirochaetal infection due to *Treponema pertenue*. This spirochaete is indistinguishable morphologically from *Treponema pallidum*, the cause of syphilis.

(c) In early childhood, probably by direct contact with a skin lesion on his mother.

(d) At this advanced stage the organism cannot be found in the lesions. There are marked radiological changes, but these vary greatly. Treponemal serology is positive. After this long time the reaginic tests may be negative but the specific tests, such as the TPHA and FTA.Abs, will be positive. They do not distinguish between yaws and syphilis.

(e) Yes, by treatment of the early disease with penicillin. In the late 1950s mass campaigns, using small doses of penicillin, virtually eradicated yaws from the humid topics.

29 (a) Q fever. Pneumonitis is a common manifestation.

(b) Yes. Human infection is derived from infected animals such as cattle, sheep or goats. The placenta and other products of conception may be highly infectious.

(c) *Coxiella burnetii*.

(d) From 2 to 4 weeks.

30 (a) An egg of *Schistosoma mansoni*; note the lateral spine.

(b) Eggs hatch in water, releasing miracidia, which enter freshwater snails. Cercariae released from snails penetrate the skin of man and, after migration, adult flukes come to lie in the venous plexus surrounding the bowel, where eggs are laid.

(c) Yes. Intestinal schistosomiasis may give rise to portal hypertension.

(d) Eggs, carried embolically from the gut to the liver via the portal vein, result in the formation of granulomata and subsequent fibrosis in the portal tracts, leading to portal hypertension. Splenomegaly and oesophageal varices follow.

(e) Children tolerate haematemesis well. Since there is initially comparatively little liver cell damage, liver failure is not an early feature. The long-term prognosis, however, is not good.

31 (a) Kaposi's sarcoma. There is a European variant with a peak incidence in the sixth and seventh decades of life, and an African one with a peak in the third decade.
(b) By biopsy.
(c) HIV causing acquired immune deficiency syndrome (AIDS).
(d) The gastro-intestinal tract is the main site of spread. Lymphoreticular neoplasia develops in 10 per cent of patients with the European variety, but is uncommon in patients with the African variety.

32 (a) Trophozoites of *Plasmodium vivax*; the parasitised cells are enlarged and Schüffner's dots are present.
(b) The parasitaemia is much higher than usually found. About 5 per cent of the red blood cells are parasitised, whereas parasitaemia is usually less than 1 per cent.
(c) Yes. Vivax malaria is a relapsing infection.
(d) This will bring the current attack to an end but may not be curative, since even the best schizontocides will not eradicate the exoerythrocytic forms of the parasite, which are responsible for relapses.
(e) Apart from relapse there are no sequelae of a vivax infection.

33 (a) A rash emerging after the temperature has returned to normal is typical of roseola infantum. If the child has been given treatment with antibiotics the rash mistakenly may be thought to be caused by drug hypersensitivity.
(b) Probably a virus infection, although this has not been identified.
(c) Between 10 and 15 days.
(d) Convulsions are common at the onset of illness, but other complications are rare.

34 (a) The history and appearance suggest Buruli ulcer.
(b) Even when extensive this infection characteristically involves superficial structures only, and bone is not involved.
(c) Extension of the lesion can involve very large areas, such as a whole upper limb.
(d) Not at this stage; at a later stage discharge may be caused by secondary infection.
(e) Biopsy will show the characteristic histology, namely superfical necrosis and the presence of acid-fast bacilli. Culture will yield *Mycobacterium ulcerans*.

35 (a) An inclusion body.
(b) Inclusion conjunctivitis of the newborn.
(c) *Chlamydia trachomatis*. Microscopy is relatively insensitive in detecting the presence of this organism, and tissue culture is preferable.
(d) The conjunctivitis may progress to mild trachoma; this is more common in older children and adults following persistent or recurrent infection.

36 (a) Extensive patchy shadowing in the right upper and mid zones.
(b) Pneumonia due to Legionnaires' disease. The slow onset and progressive course of the illness, and the severe respiratory distress in combination with diarrhoea and mental disturbance, are very suggestive. The high ESR and abnormal biochemical findings are also supportive.
(c) By demonstrating a fourfold rise in antibodies in paired sera taken 3–6 weeks apart.
(d) Yes. Older patients, especially immune deficient, are very vulnerable to hospital-acquired infection.
(e) The probable source is infected air-conditioning plant. Case-to-case spread is rare if it occurs at all.

37 (a) Marked distortion of the fauces due to oedema, and the presence of gelatinous black membrane extending over the palate.
(b) Pharyngeal diphtheria.
(c) Exotoxin produced by the diphtheria bacilli growing in the throat is absorbed and damages the heart muscle cells.
(d) Neuropathy, resulting in lower motor neurone pareses.

38 (a) Rods with terminal spherical spores characteristic of *Clostridium tetani*. The culture was made anaerobically.
(b) It is frequently found in the intestinal tract of animals and sometimes of man. It is especially prevalent where there is cow or horse manure.
(c) It is likely that many wounds are contaminated with *C. tetani* and that clinical tetanus may not develop even in the non-immunised.
(d) He should be protected by immunisation. If there is any doubt about immunity he should be given antitetanus serum followed by active immunisation with toxoid.
(e) Clinical tetanus is unusual following antitetanus serum or in those fully immunised with toxoid. Should it develop, it may be less severe than in the non-immune, but still carries a mortality rate.

39 (a) Infection with *Echinococcus granulosa*, producing a hydatid cyst.
(b) Scolices and daughter cells.
(c) Yes. In view of the presenting symptoms, the purpose of the exploration was to remove the cyst.
(d) Care must be taken not to spill the cyst contents into the peritoneal cavity, because this may result in the formation of multiple cysts and subsequent management may be unsatisfactory.
(e) No. Other cysts concurrently present in the liver would be detected by ultrasonic scanning unless they are very small.

40 (a) Many small opacities due to calcification.
(b) Varicella. Tuberculosis may result in widespread calcification of the lungs, but is usually not so diffuse. Measles and pertussis do not result in pulmonary calcification, whereas varicella in adult life may do so. Histoplasmosis does not occur in the UK.
(c) Varicella pneumonia is an interstitial pneumonia with numerous small foci (3 mm) of fibrinoid necrosis. Calcium salts may be deposited in these necrotic areas during healing.
(d) Excellent. The nurse had no respiratory symptoms or signs.

41 (a) Quinsy or peritonsillar abscess.
(b) In most untreated cases the abscess will point and discharge.
(c) *Streptococcus pyogenes* and anaerobic bacteria.
(d) The anginose variety of acute infectious monomucleosis occasionally may be complicated by a quinsy.

42 (a) Irido-cyclitis. The eye is inflamed, the cornea hazy, the pupil irregular.
(b) The inflamed iris adheres to the posterior surface of the cornea.
(c) A heavy rash on the side of the nose is a warning that the naso-ciliary branch of the ophthalmic division is severely affected and irido-cyclitis a strong possibility.
(d) Adhesions may be prevented by dilating the pupil with a mydriatic at an early stage of the illness.

43 (a) It has the characteristic wheel-like appearance of a rotavirus. This virus belongs to the family *Reoviridae* and has a double capsid containing double-stranded RNA. Two serotypes have been indentified in humans.
(b) Fever and vomiting, followed by diarrhoea. This frequently leads to dehydration.
(c) In the USA most children have serological evidence of infection by 3 years of age.
(d) Adults may become infected, but seldom develop gastro-enteritis.

44 (a) Tinea imbricata, other forms of tinea and icthyosis. The absence of marked inflammation, the large size of the scales and the concentric rings favour tinea imbricata rather than other forms of tinea, as does the distribution of the eruption. The concentric arrangement of the scales and, on closer inspection, their peripheral attachment are points against a diagnosis of icthyosis. Detection of abundant fungus in the skin would confirm the diagnosis of tinea imbricata.
(b) *Trichophyton concentricum*.
(c) An even, warm temperature and high humidity favour this infection. Regular oiling of the skin affords some protection.

45 (a) Diffuse fine nodular shadowing.
(b) The preceding history and the subacute course of the respiratory infection point to a diagnosis of pneumocystis or cytomegalovirus pneumonia.
(c) Acquired immune deficiency syndrome.
(d) Only by demonstrating the organism in material obtained from the respiratory tract by endotracheal brush technique, or by open lung biopsy or by percutaneous needle aspiration. Cytomegalovirus may be cultured from the respiratory secretions or blood.
(e) Human immunodeficiency virus (HIV).

46 (a) A microfilaria of *Wuchereria bancrofti*; the nuclei stop short of the tip of the tail and the parasite is sheathed.
(b) The infection is spread from man to man by bites of various mosquitoes.
(c) The adult filariae live within lymphatics and when they die a host response is mounted against them. Granulomata are formed around the worms and there is also an intermediate type hypersensitivity component.
(d) Chyluria. The presence of intestinal lymph in the urine is a feature of the infection in some parts of the world. In males the external genitalia may be involved in the inflammatory response seen in this patient.
(e) Untreated, the acute attack will subside but is likely to recur. Eventually lymphoedema persists between attacks and elephantoid changes then develop.

47 (a) Strabismus and conjunctivitis.
(b) Third nerve palsy due to herpes zoster. Note the pigmentation and scarring over the forehead and nose, caused by herpes zoster of the fifth cranial nerve.
(c) Most patients with external ophthalmoplegia due to herpes zoster recover completely over 3–6 months.

48 (a) Oriental sore, the cutaneous form of leishmaniasis due to protozoa *Leishmania tropica*.
(b) From the domestic dog to man by the bite of the sandfly, *Phlebotomus* spp.
(c) By aspiration from the edge of the lesion to demonstrate the amastigote of leishmania.
(d) Infection remains localised to the skin.
(e) Over a period of months or years the lesion will heal with scarring and disfigurement, partly as a result of secondary infection.

49 (a) Kawasaki disease. The diagnosis is based on the combination of the clinical features and the course of the illness.
(b) During the recovery stage characteristic desquamation starts round the nail folds and spreads to the adjacent areas of skin.
(c) Coronary artery aneurysm, which may result in thrombosis and myocardial infarcation.
(d) The platelet count is usually markedly elevated.

50 (a) Tinea pedis which may present in three distinct clinical forms. The hyperkeratotic variety is shown, with fine to coarse scaling and minimal inflammation, usually involving the plantar surface of the foot. The most common affects the skin between the fourth and fifth toes with maceration and fissuring of the skin; less common is the vesiculo-pustular variety presenting with itchy, deep-seated blisters containing clear fluid. These may rupture and become secondarily infected.
(b) Keratophilic dermatophytes, including *Trichophyton rubra*, *T. mentagrophytes* and *T. floccosum*.
(c) Minor trauma or occlusion of the skin is necessary for the initial invasion by the fungus. Infection is confined to the stratum corneum.

51 (a) There is marked destruction of the second lumbar vertebra with loss of the intervertebral space, and also gallstones.
(b) Osteomyelitis.
(c) Patients with sickle-cell disease are especially prone to infection. Although they may occasionally develop salmonella osteomyelitis, staphylococcal infection is more common and was the cause here.
(d) Osteomyelitis is not a frequent occurrence in patients with sickle-cell disease. Gallstones are found in about 25 per cent of sickle-cell patients by the age of 20 years.
(e) The prognosis of the osteomyelitis is quite good. Under hygienic living conditions infection in patients with sickle-cell disease can be reduced so that more reach adult life.

52 (a) The appearances are typical of a herpesvirus. There is a central capsid with surface capsomeres and an outer envelope.
(b) DNA.
(c) Varicella/zoster, herpes simplex, infectious mononucleosis and cytomegalovirus disease.
(d) Varicella or herpes simplex.

53 (a) A parasite cut across in two places and surrounded by fibrous tissue.
(b) Yes. The parasite is the helminth *Onchocerca volvulus*. The host response against the microfilariae is responsible for the irritating rash.
(c) Yes. Skin snips, especially if taken from the shoulders, buttocks or calves, show microfilariae.
(d) A major host response is an immediate type hypersensitivity reaction against dead or damaged microfilariae. Thus, treatment especially effective against microfilariae often increases symptoms.
(e) Yes. Interstitial keratitis with or without retinal lesions may lead to blindness. Again, the host response is against microfilariae dying in the cornea.

54 (a) Chancroid. The rather ragged appearance, apparent fusion of individual lesions to form a larger lesion, lack of induration, and the tenderness of the ulcer and inguinal gland all indicate chancroid.
(b) The organism responsible, *Haemophilus ducreyi*, may be seen on smear or isolated on culture of a swab from the ulcer or of aspirate from the gland.
(c) Dark-field examination of the exudate from the ulcer and serological tests for syphilis should be carried out since syphilis coexists in 10 per cent of patients with chancroid.

(d) Occasionally the ulcers may become secondarily infected, with extensive tissue destruction.

55 (a) This chronic paronychia with involvement of the nails themselves is most likely due to *Candida albicans* infection. Psoriasis may also give nail deformity, even in the absence of joint involvement.
(b) *Candida albicans* may be demonstrated in nail clippings and scrapings, especially in potassium hydroxide preparations. The organism is Gram-positive and grows readily on ordinary media.
(c) This infection occurs especially in those whose hands are frequently immersed in water, and in diabetics and those with endocrine disorders. Nail involvement as a manifestation of chronic mucocutaneous candidiasis may occur in those with immunological defects.
(d) It is chronic and refractory to treatment.
(e) Although chronic, it tends to remain confined to the nails.

56 (a) Herpes zoster, involving the first division of the fifth cranial nerve.
(b) Chemosis—oedema of the conjunctiva.
(c) Oedema of the eyelids is a common finding in herpes ophthalmicus but chemosis is much less common. Both resolve spontaneously as the acute stage subsides.
(d) She is likely to have hypoaesthesia or even anaesthesia.

57 (a) Soft nodular shadowing throughout both lungs.
(b) The findings are consistent with varicella pneumonia. This is caused by the virus, not by secondary bacterial invasion.
(c) Histological examination would reveal widely disseminated interstitial pneumonia with patchy haemorrhagic consolidation. The alveoli would be filled with protein-rich fluid containing red cells and mononuclear cells, some of which may contain typical intranuclear inclusions.
(d) It is extremely rare in children. The common pneumonia found in children with varicella is staphylococcal.

58 (a) Cutaneous anthrax. The site of the lesion, its appearance and the absence of pain are characteristic.
(b) Anthrax of the neck is an occupational hazard for hide porters.
(c) *Bacillus anthracis*, a Gram-positive sporing bacillus.
(d) Polymorphonuclear leucocytosis is the rule.
(e) This has not been reported.

59 (a) Typhoid or paratyphoid fever. Coughing is common during the first week.
(b) A rose-spot rash. In this patient it is usually heavy.
(c) Blood culture. Stool culture would not differentiate a case from a carrier and the Widal test is not reliable in every case.
(d) Ulceration of Peyer's patches may result in haemorrhage or perforation.

60 (a) A trophozoite of *Entamoeba histolytica* with some red cells, but no cellular exudate.
(b) No. A diagnosis of amoebic colitis can be made.
(c) It is likely that there will be spontaneous remission, perhaps followed by relapse. There is always the danger of large bowel perforation. Liver abscess may follow amoebic colitis, but may be found in patients with no history to suggest amoebic colitis.
(d) Post-dysenteric colitis, a condition similar to ulcerative colitis, is a rare sequela.
(e) Ingestion of cysts of *E. histolytica*, usually from water.

61 (a) Erythema nodosum.
(b) It may follow sensitisation to a number of infectious agents. Infection of the bowel with *Yersinia enterocolitica* not uncommonly causes abdominal pain and diarrhoea followed by erythema nodosum.
(c) Some patients have a rash on hands and forearms as well as on the legs.
(d) It evolves over a period of 3–4 weeks from erythematous nodules to brownish pigmentation of the skin.

62 (a) Multiple small soft infiltrates throughout both lung fields. There may be some hilar enlargement, and there is marked scoliosis convex to the right.
(b) This includes tuberculosis, toxoplasmosis, hypersensitivity pneumonitis, sarcoidosis, pulmonary eosinophilia and histoplasmosis.
(c) The complement-fixation test for histoplasmosis was positive at 1:8 on the first sample and 1:32 2 weeks later.
(d) Good. The majority of such patients recover spontaneously over a period of about 3 weeks.
(e) As the patient improves the pulmonary infiltrates will disappear. A proportion may calcify and remain as evidence of previous infection.

63 (a) Herpes simplex.
(b) *Herpesvirus hominis*—usually type 2.
(c) Radiculitis and meningitis are associated with type 2 virus infections.
(d) Infection of the genital tract with herpes virus is commonly asymptomatic in the male, but usually results in genital lesions in the female.

64 (a) Secondary syphilis.
(b) The patient may give a history of having had a chancre 2–8 weeks previously, and sometimes this may persist into the secondary stage of the disease.
(c) Lesions on mucous membranes are highly infectious.
(d) By serological tests. Reaginic tests, using non-specific cardiolipid antigen, are useful for indicating activity of the disease. Specific tests, using treponemal antigen, are used for confirmation of the diagnosis.

65 (a) Gas gangrene. Pain is an early feature and the formation of large blebs containing fluid is a characteristic finding. The degree of erythema is unusual.
(b) *Clostridium perfringens*.
(c) Gas in muscles and fascial planes.
(d) Bacteraemia is found in 15 per cent of patients and, when severe, may result in intravascular haemolysis.

66 (a) The skin lesions are characteristic of early yaws.
(b) Periostitis of the small bones of the hand.
(c) Blood culture would be sterile.
(d) Person-to-person transmission may occur by close physical contact, as between mother and infant, or perhaps mechanically by flies. Isolation is not practical or necessary.
(e) Dark-field examination of the thin exudate from the skin lesion will demonstrate *Treponema pertenue*, and treponemal serological tests will be positive.

67 (a) Pyrexia of this duration suggests typhoid fever, tuberculosis, brucellosis, bacterial endocarditis, visceral leishmaniasis or an abscess.
(b) The bone marrow smear shows many amastigotes of *Leishmania donovani* within a macrophage. The moderate pancytopenia and splenomegaly are characteristic for this duration of symptoms in visceral leishmaniasis.

(c) In India organisms may sometimes be isolated from the blood. In the Sudan diagnosis is often made by examination of the aspirate from an enlarged gland. In all endemic areas aspirate from the spleen shows parasites, although most physicians prefer marrow aspiration.

(d) Yes. Untreated visceral leishmaniasis carries almost 100 per cent mortality.

68 (a) Herpes simplex.

(b) Yes. Primary attacks in children may involve skin at any site, the mouth and occasionally the eye.

(c) *Herpesvirus hominis* type 1.

(d) It may be difficult to differentiate extensive herpes simplex infection from herpes zoster involving part of a dermatome. Mild sensory disturbance may be present in herpes simplex, but there is usually a more definite prodromal period of paraesthesia and a pain in zoster. The rashes may look similar.

69 (a) She has diffuse swelling of the parotid gland. The fever and the associated polymorphonuclear leucocytosis point to a diagnosis of suppurative parotitis.

(b) Redness of the overlying skin is an early feature. Later there may be fluctuation of the swelling. Drops of pus may be expressed from the parotid papilla.

(c) Suppurative parotitis is seen more frequently in debilitated elderly patients with dryness of the mouth and poor oral hygiene. Dryness of the mouth during and following the operation may have predisposed to spread of infection along the parotid duct.

(d) In this case the pus gave a heavy growth of *Staphylococcus aureus*.

70 (a) Multiple small cavities in the liver.

(b) Liver abscesses or multiple hydatid cysts. The short duration and severity of the symptoms favour liver abscess. In patients from that area amoebic infection would be the most probable cause.

(c) An elevated white blood cell count, high ESR, abnormal chest X-ray and positive amoebic serology would indicate amoebic liver abscess; a normal white blood cell count and sedimentation rate, a normal chest X-ray and positive hydatid serology would favour hydatid cyst.

(d) An amoebic liver abscess, if untreated, may enlarge and rupture through the abdominal wall, through the diaphragm or into the peritoneal cavity or pericardial sac.

71 (a) Bacterial urinary tract infection, polyposis and urinary schistosomiasis.

(b) Urinary tract infection is unlikely in view of the negative microscopy and culture. A polyp would be seen on cystoscopy.

(c) It shows ova of *Schistosoma haematobium*.

(d) During the passage of ova from the vesicular veins into the bladder lumen some blood also escapes; bladder contraction makes the haematuria typically terminal.

(e) This usually follows treatment unless there has been reduced renal function as a result of hydronephrosis or there is malignant change.

72 (a) Acute infectious mononucleosis with an ampicillin-induced rash.

(b) Clinically, it may be suspected by detecting splenomegaly and generalised lymphadenopathy. It is confirmed by demonstrating a high proportion of atypical mononuclear cells in the peripheral blood and by detecting heterophil antibodies against sheep or horse red blood cells.

(c) About two-thirds of patients with infectious mononucleosis given ampicillin will develop a drug-induced rash.

73 (a) Cysts of *Entamoeba histolytica*. These measure 10–12 μm and show the characteristic chromidial bar and nuclei.
(b) No.
(c) Not if he is now asymptomatic and has not had diarrhoea recently. It is known that many strains of *E. histolytica* are non-pathogenic.
(d) The natural history of amoebic infection is not known precisely. It is likely that the cysts will disappear from his stools over the next few weeks or months.
(e) Amoebic infection is acquired by ingesting cysts. The patient is, therefore, a source of infection but transmission is less likely where the standard of hygiene is high.

74 (a) Splinter haemorrhages.
(b) Infective endocarditis.
(c) Vasculitis due to deposition of immune complexes. Splinter haemorrhages were formerly attributed to micro-emboli.
(d) Cardiac murmur; embolism; splenomegaly.

75 (a) Leprosy.
(b) The weakness and deformity of the hands suggest that originally the patient was in the middle of the spectrum of disease (borderline). The pale areas of the back are characteristic of lepromatous leprosy, suggesting that he has recently moved towards that end of the spectrum.
(c) The nodules on the limbs may be those of erythema nodosum leprosum (ENL); the swellings of the face are characteristic of leprosy and contain macrophages packed with bacilli.
(d) By split smears from lesions or from ear lobes.
(e) Lepromatous patients discharge large numbers of bacilli, especially in nasal secretions. It may be advisable to isolate him for 2 or 3 weeks, until chemotherapy has rendered him non-infectious.

76 (a) Erysipelas. This is frequently mistaken for herpes zoster; in both conditions there may be an erythematous rash with bullae. However, the rash of erysipelas appears after a few hours of discomfort and does not conform to a nerve root distribution, whereas herpes zoster has a longer prodromal period and a characteristic distribution involving a dermatone.
(b) *Streptococcus pyogenes*.
(c) The face and leg.
(d) Infected respiratory secretions of human origin.
(e) The most common complication is lymphoedema of the legs. Erysipelas of the legs may be complicated by abscess formation but this is very rare in facial erysipelas. Septicaemia is very unusual.

77 (a) Mastitis and pustular dermatitis.
(b) *Staphylococcus aureus*.
(c) Her baby. Most staphylococcal infections in babies are trivial and consist of pustules and septic bullae, particularly around the nail folds. Some neonates may be symptomless carriers of staphylococci in the nose and throat.
(d) Maternal sepsis may be the first indication of staphylococcal outbreak in a maternity unit.

78 (a) Eczema herpeticum.
(b) By demonstrating herpes virus particles on electron microscopy or by culturing the virus.
(c) Infection is derived from someone with a cold sore or from a carrier, who is shedding virus in saliva. Patients with eczema are particularly susceptible because skin immunity is defective.

(d) Infection may be spread by direct transfer of virus from one part of the skin to another or by bloodstream invasion and dissemination. In the case of systemic spread, other organs may be affected by the virus, and there may be evidence of liver or myocardial damage.

79 (a) Crimea–Congo haemorrhagic fever.
(b) A virus belonging to the *Nairovirus* genus of the *Bunyaviridae* family.
(c) By ticks, especially *Hyalomma*.
(d) Domestic animals (sheep, goats and cattle) and wild animals.

80 (a) Irregular opacities due to intracranial calcification.
(b) Congenital toxoplasmosis is responsible in 50 per cent of cases.
(c) Hydrocephalus, mental retardation, epilepsy and choroidoretinitis.
(c) Congenital infection occurs in about one-third of infants of mothers primarily infected in pregnancy; about one-third of the infected infants develop clinical disease.

81 (a) Many small rings of *Plasmodium falciparum*.
(b) The parasitaemia cannot be determined from a thick film stained in this way, since the red blood cells are destroyed.
(c) Yes. It suggests that she has some degree of renal failure, a common finding in heavy falciparum infections, due to occlusion of the renal capillaries by parasitised red blood cells in the renal capillaries.
(d) Complicated malaria, of which renal failure is a manifestation, carries a mortality if untreated. If consciousness is also impaired, late or inappropriate treatment may be unsuccessful.

82 (a) This rests between herpes simplex stomatitis and herpangina. The individual lesions are similar in both. The lesions of herpangina tend to be confined to the posterior half of the mouth, whereas those of herpes simplex tend to involve the anterior half. Herpangina is predominantly a disease of children.
(b) Herpes simplex stomatitis is usually a primary infection.
(c) By culture of the virus.
(d) Most primary attacks of herpes simplex involving the mouth are caused by *Herpesvirus hominis* type I.

83 (a) Yaws, syphilis, leprosy, mucocutaneous leishmaniasis.
(b) The mucosal lesions of mucocutaneous leishmaniasis, due to *Leishmania braziliensis* and *L. mexicana*, may be preceded by a skin lesion at the site where the sandfly, of the genus *Lutzomya*, injected the parasite.
(c) The leishmanin skin test (delayed hypersensitivity) will be postitive in previous leishmania infection; the treponemal serological tests will be positive in syphilis and yaws; the lepromin test is negative in leprosy towards the lepromatous end of the spectrum.
(d) Biopsy of the nasal mucosa should be performed.
(e) Progressive destruction of the septum should be halted by treatment.

84 (a) Carbuncle.
(b) *Staphylococcus aureus*.
(c) Diabetes mellitus is an uncommon predisposing cause, which should always be excluded.
(d) Invasion of a hair follicle gives rise to a small abscess or boil. When several adjacent hair follicles are involved the abscesses merge to form a carbuncle.

85 (a) Cysts of *Giardia lamblia*.
(b) The giardia infection may have contributed to his recent diarrhoea but is not responsible for the blood he passed previously or for the sigmoidoscopic findings.
(c) Culture of his stool for shigella and campylobacter might demonstrate a cause for the proctitis. Rectal biospy and barium enema might show the features of inflammatory bowel disease.
(d) Inflammatory bowel disease with associated giardiasis.
(e) The giardia infection can be eradicated. If inflammatory bowel disease is present it is likely to follow a benign course in this particular patient.

86 (a) Acute glomerulonephritis.
(b) Oedema from fluid retention, hypertension and uraemia.
(c) A nephritogenic strain of *Streptococcus pyogenes*.
(d) Yes. Nephritogenic strains are more common in the tropics, where nephritis is commonly associated with streptococcal infection of the skin.
(e) Most children recover completely.

87 (a) Actinomycosis. This is caused by filamentous branching Gram-positive bacteria, the one most commonly infecting man being *Actinomyces israeli*.
(b) The most probable starting point is the mouth, especially through a tooth. Spread is then to the neck, and from there to the back. Alternatively infection in the mouth or neck may involve the lungs by aspiration and then the chest wall by direct extension.
(c) Yes. the characteristic 'sulphur granules' are yellow aggregrates of organisms cemented together by calcium phosphate of host origin.
(d) Crushed granules or discharging pus should be cultured anaerobically in thioglycollate broth.
(e) In this patient it may be expected to be normal. If the chest wall were infected by direct extension from the lung, then the chest X-ray may suggest tuberculosis or malignancy.

88 (a) Impetigo contagiosa.
(b) Impetigo may be caused by *Streptococcus pyogenes* or *Staphylococcus aureus*, or by a combination of both. The staphylococci commonly belong to phage group II and many are resistant to benzyl penicillin.
(c) Impetigo may complicate such skin conditions as pediculosis, scabies, eczema and acute fungus infections.

89 (a) The combination of symptoms points to rat-bite fever or other form of septicaemia.
(b) Rat-bite fever but there was no history of a rat bite.
(c) Blood culture gave a growth of *Streptobacillus moniliformis*.
(d) This organism can be transmitted to man by a rat bite or by drinking contaminated raw milk. When the infection is milk-borne it is designated Haverhill fever.
(e) If untreated, the illness characteristically follows a relapsing course over a period of several weeks or even months.

90 (a) Varicella.
(b) In any patient with varicella who has an unusually high or prolonged fever, blood should be cultured to exclude a septicaemia. *Staphylococcus aureus* is the common invader and was grown from this patient's cultures. The same organism was grown from the large pustule on her chin.
(c) It may be due to hepatitis caused by varicella, or may be caused by the staphylococcal septicaemia.
(d) In patients with Hodgkin's disease there is an appreciable mortality from untreated varicella. Death may result directly from the uncontrolled virus infection or from secondary bacterial invasion.

91 (a) These are target lesions of erythema multiforme and may be a component of Stevens–Johnson syndrome, The skin lesions are erythematous with
concentric rings of different colours.
(b) Various combinations of conjunctivitis, stomatitis and urethritis or vul-
vitis. Stevens–Johnson syndrome consists of the rash in combination with the
other three components.
(c) A hypersensitivity response to an infectious agent or to drugs. In many
cases the cause cannot be determined.
(d) The rash begins to fade after 10–14 days and may leave some staining.
Most patients make a complete and uneventful recovery.

92 (a) Rhabditiform larva of *Strongyloides stercoralis*.
(b) Yes. Heavy bowel infection with strongyloides may cause diarrhoea and
migrating larvae are a cause of pulmonary eosinophilia.
(c) Infective larvae in the soil penetrate the skin of man and, after migration,
develop into adult worms in the gut. Female worms are larviparous; larvae in
the stools reach the soil and the cycle is completed.
(d) There is also a cycle within man without a free-living form. In those
immunosuppressed by disease or treatment, the number of parasites may
increase greatly.
(e) Overwhelming infection in the immunosuppressed and untreated carries a
mortality.

93 (a) Measles. A prodromal stage of acute respiratory tract catarrh followed
by a maculo-papular rash evolving from above downwards is characteristic.
Note the congestion of the conjunctivae and the crusting of the nostrils.
(b) An inflamed buccal mucosa; Koplik's spots present during the prodromal
stage but fading within 24 hours of the onset of the rash.
(c) Measles virus, a paramyxovirus containing a single strand of RNA.
(d) Otitis media and secondary bacterial pneumonia. Post-measles encephalitis is a more serious complication but is relatively uncommon.

94 (a) Advanced fibroid tuberculosis with extensive fibrosis and calcification
in the right lung.
(b) It is not possible to decide from the appearance of the X-ray film.
Specimens of sputum or gastric washings should be examined for acid-fast
bacilli and cultures taken for mycobacteria.
(c) The most probable organism is *Mycobacterium tuberculosis*; 0.7-4 per cent
of patients with radiographic shadows suggestive of pulmonary tuberculosis
yield atypical mycobacteria on culture.

95 (a) Widely spaced peg-shaped upper incisors with notching (Hutchinson's
teeth).
(b) No.
(c) Stool microscopy and culture. Treponemal serology is required for the
abnormality of the teeth.
(d) Congenital syphilis results from the passage of *Treponema pallidum*
across the placenta after the 4th month of pregnancy. Infection of the mother
has usually taken place within the previous year.
(e) No. Other characteristic features are the early rhinitis, skin rash, saddle
nose and liver involvement. Interstitial keratitis and deafness may develop in
adolescence and later still arthropathy of the knees (Clutton's joints).

96 (a) This is the rural form of cutaneous lesishmaniasis. The appearance of these multiple crusted lesions with surrounding erythema and the possibility of exposure in an endemic area is characteristic. Infected insect bites do not have the crusting.

(b) The organism responsible, *Leishmania major*, is transmitted by the bite of the sandfly, *Phlebotomus*. The reservoir of infection is wild rodents.

(c) By demonstrating the amastigotes of the parasite in the aspirate taken from the edge of the lesion.

(d) The lesions will heal over a period of weeks or months.

97 (a) Embryonated hookworm egg.

(b) Hookworm infection may give rise to an iron-deficiency anaemia and the haematological results are consistent with iron deficiency.

(c) Iron deficiency results when iron stores are depleted. Treatment of the hookworm infection would remove the cause of iron loss.

(d) Administration of iron would restore the haemoglobin findings to normal, but it would be advisable also to treat the hookworm infection.

(e) Hookworms attached to the small intestinal mucosa are responsible for blood loss and hence iron loss. Haemoglobin production will be maintained while iron stores last but once they have been depleted the haemoglobin will fall.

98 (a) A diluted tubule, and the lining epithelial cells contain large intra-nuclear inclusion bodies ('Owl-eye' bodies).

(b) Cytomegalovirus—one of the herpesviruses.

(c) Congenital or perinatal infection is often asymptomatic but may give rise to serious illness with jaundice, brain damage, chorioretinitis, pneumonia and gastro-intestinal disturbance.

(d) Not only may it be transferred with the donor organ, but immunosuppressive therapy may reactivate latent virus in the recipient. Infection in most patients is asymptomatic.

(e) It may be transmitted by transfusion of fresh blood at operation. It is not transmitted by stored blood.

99 (a) There has been secondary invasion of the skin and subcutaneous tissues by a skin bacterium. This has resulted in gangrene, with subsequent sloughing of the necrotic tissues.

(b) Secondary infection of varicella lesions is usually caused by *Staphylococcus aureus* or *Streptococcus pyogenes*. In this condition the probable invader is *Staphylococcus aureus*, which produces alpha haemolysin and other toxins, causing death of cells.

(c) Invasion of the bloodstream may result in septicaemia.

(d) Extensive ulceration of this type will necessitate skin grafting, otherwise there will be severe scarring and possibly keloid formation.

100 (a) Multiple well-circumscribed opacities throughout both lung fields.

(b) Yes. Pulmonary hydatid disease.

(c) Serological tests for hydatid disease will be positive.

(d) Hydatid cyst of the lung is much less common than of the liver. When single it is thought to be blood-borne. The appearances here suggest bronchogenic spread from a single cyst which ruptured into an air passage.

(e) In the absence of chemotherapy the prognosis is poor.

101 (a) Trophozoites of *Plasmodium ovale*.

(b) *Plasmodium ovale* infections show a 48-hour periodicity, which may not develop for some days after the start of pyrexia.

(c) It is perhaps surprising that she gives no history of fever in Uganda; the symptoms may have been mild. The long asymptomatic period in Britain results from the persistence of the liver forms of the parasite (exoerythrocytic forms).

(d) It would rapidly bring to an end the current febrile illness, but further relapses may occur unless the liver forms are eradicated.

(e) Apart from relapse there are no sequelae.

102 (a) Ecthyma, a deeply ulcerated form of impetigo.

(b) Skin strains of *Streptococcus pyogenes*. *Staphylococcus aureus* may also be present but does not appear to play an active part in the disease process.

(c) Streptococcal impetigo has a peak incidence in children of 2-5 years, whereas streptococcal infections of the throat predominantly involve older children in the 5–15 year group.

(d) Poor hygiene, warm humid climate and minor trauma to the legs.

(e) Post-streptococcal nephritis. Suppurative complications are unusual and rheumatic fever does not occur.

103 (a) Cutaneous larva migrans. Itchy papules develop at the sites where the larvae enter the skin and linear streaks later mark the course of the larvae as they migrate through the epidermis.

(b) Larvae of various species of animal hookworms, such as *Ankylostoma caninum*. *A. braziliense* and *A. ceylanicum*.

(c) Sandy beaches in the tropics may be contaminated by dog faeces containing hookworm eggs. These develop into infective larvae and invade the skin of sunbathers lying directly on the sand.

104 (a) Secondary syphilis. The rash is a syphilide of papulo-squamous/pustular type and the mouth lesions are mucous patches. A primary chancre is still present in about 30 per cent of patients.

(b) It is usually diagnosed by serological tests. Reaginic tests are useful for indicating activity of disease but false-positive results may occur, so positive findings should be confirmed by specific tests. *Treponema pallidum* may be demonstrated in specimen taken from mucous patches.

(c) Mucous patches are highly infectious.

(d) Skin lesions may persist for 4–6 weeks. Enlargement of lymph nodes may take several months to subside.

105 (a) Tinea capitis of inflammatory type. In some patients this may progress to suppuration as a result of an allergic response. The lesion is then described as a kerion.

(b) Tinea capitis is caused by fungi belonging to the genera *Trichophton* or *Microsporum*.

(c) *Microsporum* infections are common in early childhood but the incidence falls sharply after 10 years of age. Most cases of inflammatory tinea capitis are caused by ectothrix infection, whereas non-inflammatory disease may be caused by either ectothrix or endothrix infection.

(d) The infected hairs in ectothrix infections can be identified by fluorescence under Wood's lamp. They can then be removed and examined microscopically in a potassium hydroxide preparation, or the fungus can be cultured.

106 (a) Collapse of the right lung and mediastinal shift to the left. There is obliteration of the right costophrenic angle.

(b) Pyopneumothorax complicating pneumonia. A subpleural abscess has ruptured into the pleural cavity.

(c) *Staphylococcus aureus*.

(d) In children staphylococcal pneumonia is usually a primary infection but may follow chickenpox, influenza and mucoviscidosis.

107 (a) Liver abscess; viral hepatitis but the size of the liver, white blood cell count and lack of jaundice are against this; hepatoma, which is unusual in a white male of this age.
(b) Elevation of the right hemidiaphragm, a small pleural effusion and some linear collapse would favour liver abscess.
(c) Ultrasonic scanning; amoebic serology; aspiration where there are few facilities.
(d) Amoebic cysts often are not found in the stools of patients with amoebic liver abscesses. However, amoebic infection is very common in the tropics and often can be coincidental.
(e) *Entamoeba histolytica*. Amoebic liver abscess is much more likely in these circumstances than bacterial liver abscess.

108 (a) Superficial ulceration may result from infection of insect bites or an abrasion. This lesion is clean and surrounded by pigmentation; it is the 'chancre' of African trypanosomiasis.
(b) By the bite of the tsetse fly, *Glossina*, which inoculates the metacyclic form of the trypanosome.
(c) Probably non-specific inflammatory changes without trypanosomes.
(d) Aspirate from the enlarged gland; a peripheral blood film will show the parasite.
(e) The acuteness of the illness and the obvious local lesion suggest the East African form of the disease, in which there is substantial mortality if untreated.

109 (a) A microfilaria of *Loa loa*; the nuclei extend to the tip of the tail and the parasite is sheathed.
(b) The infection is transmitted from man to man by the bite of horse flies (tabanids).
(c) An additional, or the only symptom may be an adult worm, measuring several centimetres, crossing the eye beneath the conjunctiva.
(d) Some patients may show one or both characteristic symptoms but microfilariae may not be found on repeated blood examination. There is, however, the usual eosinophilia and a positive serological test for filaria.
(e) Excellent. Following the eradication of the parasite by treatment, there are no sequelae.

110 (a) Dumb rabies.
(b) In 80 per cent of patients, following the prodrome of malaise, fever and anorexia, there is hyperactivity with periods of agitation, biting and other abnormal behaviour, followed by paralysis and coma. In 20 per cent of patients, paralysis develops without the hyperactive or 'furious' phase. This is known as 'dumb' rabies.
(c) Rabies virus may be isolated from urine, saliva or cerebrospinal fluid early in the illness. It may be demonstrated also by fluorescence in corneal smears.
(d) Rabies, whether furious or dumb, is almost 100 per cent fatal.
(e) There have been a few reports of recovery from rabies in patients who have received pre- or post-exposure vaccine and who have been ventilated.

111 (a) A peeling strawberry tongue. The fur separates from the tip and edges of the tongue, eventually leaving a red strawberry appearance.
(b) Scarlet fever.
(c) Rheumatic fever or acute nephritis may develop during the second or third week.
(d) A strain of *Streptococcus pyogenes*, producing erythrogenic toxin.

112 (a) Fine nodular shadows throughout both lungs.
(b) Miliary tuberculosis.
(c) The tuberculin test is usually strongly positive and tubercle bacilli may be grown from gastric washings. Liver biopsy may reveal characteristic granulomas.
(d) There may be signs of meningitis and tubercles may be detected in the choroid.

113 (a) Neonatal tetanus.
(b) Through the stump of the umbilical cord which in this case was cut with an unsterilised kitchen knife.
(c) Immunisation of the mother during pregnancy with tetanus toxoid gives almost complete protection to the neonate, especially if two doses are given. It could have been prevented also by proper cutting of the umbilical cord.
(d) Yes. Antitetanus serum, sedatives and antibiotic.
(e) Despite treatment, mortality is often more than 50 per cent.

114 (a) Erysipelo-cellulitis. The border of the inflamed area is less sharply defined than in pure erysipelas.
(b) *Streptococcus haemolyticus*, Lancefield group A.
(c) Damage to lymph vessels during the initial attack may result in lymphoedema, which predisposes to further infection and progressive damage. Minor trauma to the skin may facilitate invasion by the streptococcus.
(d) Local abscess formation; lymphoedema; very rarely septicaemia.

115 (a) Hand, foot and mouth disease.
(b) Coxsackie viruses types A16, A10 and A5.
(c) There is very little discomfort.
(d) Infection spreads readily within schools and family groups.

116 (a) Dilatation of renal calyces and calcification of the bladder.
(b) Microscopy of the urine might show ova of *Schistosoma haematobium*.
(c) Biopsy of rectal mucosa often shows ova in urinary schistosomiasis. Cystoscopy might show the characteristic 'sandy patches' and bladder biopsy demonstrate ova.
(d) Fibrosis in granulomata around ova in the bladder and lower ureter causes obstruction and hydronephrosis.
(e) Cercariae released from freshwater snails penetrate the skin of man.

117 (a) Both kidneys and suprarenal glands.
(b) The upper poles of the kidneys are surmounted by extensive clots at the location of the suprarenal glands.
(c) Waterhouse–Friderichsen syndrome.
(d) Septicaemia, usually due to *Neisseria meningitidis*.

118 (a) Perforating ulcer of the foot.
(b) It is found especially in tabes dorsalis, leprosy and diabetes.
(c) No, there is no features characteristic of any of the causes.
(d) Positive treponemal serology would indicate past treponemal infection.
(e) Biopsy of a thickened nerve or of a skin lesion elsewhere would almost certainly establish a diagnosis of leprosy.

119 (a) Elephantiasis.
(b) Lymphatic obstruction.
(c) Filariasis, inguinal gland removal, radiation to pelvis.

120 (a) Diffuse nodular shadows in both lungs, particularly the right, and a large thin-walled cavity on the right.

(b) Yes. The cavity is a pneumatocele and is a common feature of severe staphylococcal pneumonia in children.

(c) No. Bacterial pneumonia is a feature of the early granulocytopenic period after transplant. Between recovery of circulating granulocytes usually 20–30 days after transplant, and only 100 viral and protozoal infections predominate

(d) Cytomegalovirus and other virus infection; *Pneumocystis carinii*. In this child the cause was cytomegalovirus.

121 (a) Trophozoite (ring form) and gametocyte (crescent) of *Plasmodium falciparum*.

(b) Yes. She has trophozoites in her blood.

(c) It could have been due to malaria as the presence of gametocytes suggests that she acquired a malarial infection some time ago.

(d) Yes. Gametocytes are the sexual forms of the parasite, which are infectious to biting female mosquitoes.

(e) No. The immunity, which develops, is a slow process requiring continuing exposure to infection.

122 (a) In an Asian patient a swelling of this type probably would be an enlarged lymph node, caused by tuberculosis.

(b) Tuberculous glands may be found at a number of superficial sites, although a single gland is more common.

(c) Especially in Asian patients, mediastinal glandular involvement may be associated with superficial tuberculous glands.

(d) A negative tuberculin test would virtually exclude tuberculosis. A positive result would be of little value, since a high proportion of adult Indians are tuberculin-positive. A strongly positive result, epecially if there were ulceration, would indicate a tuberculous origin.

(e) By a biopsy. Granulomata with caseation are virtually diagnostic of tuberculosis. Acid-fast bacilli are not often demonstrated in the tissue but *Mycobacterium tuberculosis* may be grown.

123 (a) Reiter's disease.

(b) Keratoderma blenorrhagica. The rash is commonly confined to the soles of the feet, but in severe cases may extend to other parts of the body. Lesions of the penis are found in about 25 per cent of cases.

(c) It may be found in association with sexually-transmitted non-specific urethritis, or with bacillary or amoebic dysentery or non-specific diarrhoea.

(d) Iritis may appear months or years after the onset of the disease and may result in blindness.

124 (a) A subconjunctival haemorrhage.

(b) Whooping cough. This should be suspected whenever a child has a spasmodic cough terminating in a bout of vomiting.

(c) It is primarily clinical. In a proportion of patients *Bordetella pertussis* may be isolated from a pernasal swab or from a cough plate. A white blood cell count frequently shows an absolute lymphocytosis.

(d) The blood eventually will be absorbed completely and there will be no residual damage. Until the blood is absorbed it will remain bright red because of diffusion of oxygen across the conjunctiva.

125 (a) Solices of *Echinococcus granulosa* showing hooklets and, less clearly, suckers.

(b) The chest pain was caused by the hydatid cyst seen on X-ray. Rupture of the cyst into a bronchus resulted in the expectoration of the cyst contents including solices, which are the developing parasites.

(c) Since 90 per cent of hydatid cysts are found in the liver it would be advisable to carry out an ultrasonic scan of the liver.

(d) Rupture of a hyatid cyst may result in an immediate type hypersensitivity reaction. In this patient an erythematous rash, bronchospasm and hypotension may have resulted.

126 (a) Yes. Contrast medium has travelled from the para-aortic lymphatics outwards towards the kidneys and some calyces are outlined.

(b) Milky urine.

(c) Chyluria resulting from Bancroftian filariasis.

127 (a) Intranuclear inclusion bodies are present in some of the cells. An unstained halo separates the inclusion from the nuclear membrane. Some of the cells show evidence of impending necrosis and may be recognised by their pyknotic nuclei.

(b) Disseminated herpes infection.

(c) Spread of infection from the mother's genital tract at birth or from an attendant. *Herpesvirus hominis*, type 2, is found in 80 per cent of cases.

(d) If herpetic lesions are present in the mother's genital tract at birth, about 40 per cent of neonates will be infected. The risk of severe infection in the neonate is greater in primary infection of the mother than in recurrent infection.

128 (a) He has had a septicaemia.

(b) Gangrene of his toes.

(c) In a young person this is most likely to have been caused by either *Neisseria meningitidis* or *Staphylococcus aureus*.

(d) Thrombosis of arteries or arterioles paradoxically may be associated with disseminated intravascular coagulation (DIC).

129 (a) Yes. These are trypanosomes and are probably the cause of the illness.

(b) No.

(c) Trypanosomiasis contracted in this part of the tropics often involves the nervous system early. A lumbar puncture, therefore, should be performed.

(d) One of the skin lesions may develop into the characteristic 'chancre'. Circinate skin lesions, splenomegaly and anaemia may appear.

(e) Poor, since involvement of the nervous system may occur early.

130 (a) Cutaneous larva migrans.

(b) An urticarial lesion on the skin of the buttocks is probably caused by migration of larvae of *Strongyloides stercoralis*.

(c) By demonstrating larvae in the stool or in duodenal fluid.

(d) Autoinfection with larvae of *Strongyloides stercoralis* in the immunocompromised host may result in massive invasion of the lungs and other organs, causing severe illness and even death.

131 (a) There are intra-epithelial vesicles and multinucleated giant cells.

(b) The appearances are consistent with the vesicles of varicella, herpes zoster or herpes simplex.

(c) Either *Herpesvirus hominis* or *Herpesvirus varicellae/zoster*.

132 (a) Congenital rubella.

(b) Rubella virus may be cultured from urine or throat secretions for up to 18 months after birth. Active infection in the infant may be confirmed by demonstrating rubella-specific antibody in IgM or an increase of rubella antibody in IgG on serial testing.

(c) The highest incidence of purpura occurs in infants infected between the 4th-8th weeks of pregnancy.

(d) Purpura is commonly associated with other serious defects. A high proportion have hepatomegaly, splenomegaly, congenital heart disease and eye defects.

(e) Mortality is about 30 per cent. In surviving infants the platelet count returns to normal within 1-4 months.

133 (a) Liver.
(b) Granuloma around an amorphous mass.
(c) Schistomiasis.
(d) *Schistosoma mansoni* ova.
(e) Yes. Continued egg deposition may lead to irreversible portal fibrosis.

134 (a) Clinically he had endocarditis involving the aortic valve. Damage to the valve was progressive and possibly culminated with rupture followed by pulmonary oedema.

(b) Repeatedly negative blood cultures in a patient with left-sided endocarditis suggests an infection by organisms other than bacteria commonly responsible for endocarditis. Thus *coxiella* or *histoplasma* should be considered.

(c) *Coxiella* usually infects abnormal valves, most commonly affected is the aortic valve. This patient had a bicuspid aortic valve.

(d) In patients with coxiella endocarditis the complement-fixation test is strongly positive to phase I antigen. The section shows nest of coxiella organisms.

(e) Infection is derived from animals, especially cattle, sheep and goats.

135 (a) A stye or hordeleum, which is an infected sebaceous gland on an eyelid.
(b) Usually *Staphylococcus aureus*.
(c) The nasal vestibule.
(d) Recurring styes are associated with persistent nasal carriage in the patient, or the presence of a carrier within the household.

136 (a) A wedge-shaped deformity of two vertebral bodies with narrowing of the disc space below but little formation of new bone. There is radio-opaque material in the subarachnoid space.

(b) Tuberculosis; brucellosis; hyatid disease, which is common in Cyprus.

(c) The fact that contrast medium has been introduced suggests that he has symptoms of cord compression.

(d) Exploration necessary to make a definitive diagnosis, especially of hydatid disease. Serological tests are not entirely reliable.

137 (a) Mumps involving the parotid glands.
(b) A paramyxovirus containing RNA.
(c) During the latter part of the incubation period, for several days before the parotitis appears and for several days afterwards. Regarded infectious until the swelling has subsided.
(d) It is elevated in 70 per cent of patients, irrespective of the clinical syndrome.

138 (a) Nest of amastigotes of *Trypanosoma cruzi*, the protozoon parasite responsible for Chagas' disease.

(b) No. The mortality in the acute phase of the disease is 5–10 per cent.

(c) On clinical examination the eye swelling (Romana's sign) is highly characteristic. During the acute phase trypanosomes may be found in the peripheral blood film and also by xenodiagnosis, when bugs responsible for the transmission of the disease are fed on the patient and the gut examined for trypanosomes after several weeks. Serological tests are also available.

(d) The acute illness would have subsided after a variable period and the features of Chagas' disease probably would not have developed. A history of acute illness is unusual in patients with Chagas' disease.

139 (a) The presence of a herald patch preceding the main eruption is diagnostic of pityriasis rosea.
(b) Slight redness of the throat and minimal enlargement of the cervical lymph nodes, but general disturbance is trivial.
(c) For 4–8 weeks from onset.
(d) It is most unusual to recognise case-to-case transmission.

140 (a) There is miliary shadowing throughout both lung fields.
(b) Tuberculosis, pulmonary eosinophilia, histoplasmosis, toxoplasmosis and hypersensitivity pneumonitis.
(c) The high dye-test titre points to a diagnosis of acquired toxoplamosis. The X-ray changes may be due to this infection. The absence of constitutional upset weighs against a diagnosis of miliary tuberculosis. The mild eosinophilia is related to the hookworm infection.
(d) Good.
(e) Pregnancy is not advisable while she has active toxoplasmosis, although with such a dye-test titre foetal infection would be unlikely.

141 (a) Destruction of the nose and hard palate.
(b) Leprosy (as in this patient) or syphilis.
(c) It may be apparent from the history and other physical signs. Leprosy may be confirmed by slit-skin smears and by histology of skin or nerve lesions. Syphilis may be established by specific serological tests. False-positive reaginic tests for treponema may be found in lepromatous leprosy.

142 (a) Toxic-shock syndrome.
(b) The vagina. It is usually associated with the use of tampons during menstruation.
(c) *Staphylococcus aureus*, producing enterotoxin F.

143 (a) An enterovirus infection with either ECHO virus or Coxsackie virus. The absence of respiratory symptoms or signs is against a diagnosis of measles. Rubella is a possibility, although the rash is rather scanty and coarse for this diagnosis.
(b) An ECHO virus a Coxsackie virus.
(c) In faeces or in throat secretions.
(d) Aseptic meningitis, respiratory and enteric disease.

144 (a) Aspiration of the liver.
(b) To diagnose liver abscess.
(c) Probably elevation of the right hemidiaphragm; perhaps, a small pleural effusion with some linear collapse at the base.
(d) Ultrasonic scan and amoebic serology.
(e) Amoebic liver abscess and the aspirated material is characteristic.

145 (a) This is a lymph gland stained by Ziehl–Neelson's method and shows acid-fast bacilli.
(b) Since he has always lived in India, his tuberculin test would be expected to be positive. If the test site ulcerated this would favour a tuberculous aetiology for the swelling of the neck.
(c) A chest X-ray probably will be normal. If he were febrile and unwell the X-ray might also show enlarged mediastinal glands.
(d) Either by drinking milk containing *Mycobacterium bovis* or by inhaling *M. tuberculosis*.
(e) No, he is not infectious provided that he does not have a discharging sinus and there is no evidence of active pulmonary disease.

146 (a) The X-ray appearances are those of chronic osteomyelitis with bone destruction surrounded by sclerosis. Gas can be seen subcutaneously.
(b) Bacterial culture of the discharge is unlikely to be helpful.
(c) Infection with the fungus *Madurella mycetomi*; culture on Sabourand's medium may demonstrate the organism.
(d) Slow local spread is likely; metastatic spread is most unusual.
(e) It is thought that a puncture wound carries the organism from the soil. Infection beginning in the thigh is unusual.

147 (a) These are the early framboesial lesions of yaws.
(b) Similar lesions continue to appear while older lesions resolve without scarring.
(c) Yes, especially of long bones. The lesion is a periostitis.
(d) No.
(e) The clinical appearance is highly characteristic. Dark-field examination of the exudate from the skin lesions will show the spirochaete *Treponema pertenue*, and treponemal serological tests will be positive.

148 (a) A corneal ulcer.
(b) The attack of herpes zoster has resulted in anaesthesia of the cornea, and mechanical trauma has abraided the surface.
(c) The most serious one is perforation of the anterior chamber. Ulceration may result in corneal scarring.
(d) The cornea should be protected by wearing a pad or, in severe and resistant ulceration, by performing a tarsorraphy.

149 (a) Pigment.
(b) Malarial infection.
(c) He probably suffered febrile attacks from early childhood but the immunity which develops with prolonged exposure may have rendered these mild and short-lived.
(d) No.
(e) Yes. Malaria suppression, by keeping malaria infection at a subclinical level, would have prevented this accumulation of malaria pigment.

150 (a) Koplik's spots. These are often prominent opposite the molar teeth. They are present during the prodromal stage of measles and disappear as the exanthem emerges. They may be found on any mucosal surface.
(b) Measles. Koplik's spots are pathognomonic.
(c) Appendicitis is twice as common in measles as it is in control groups. Referred pain from diaphragmatic pleurisy complicating pneumonia is more common at a later stage, when the rash has emerged. Chest X-ray is helpful in doubtful cases.
(d) No. Appendicitis in measles is associated with hyperplasia of the lymph follicles and commonly proceeds to obstruction and gangrene.

151 (a) Yes. This is the eschar of tick typhus or tick-bite fever, caused by *Rickettsia conori* and transmitted by hard ticks.
(b) At the site of a bite.
(c) Cutaneous leishmaniasis caused by *Leishmania*; Buruli ulcer caused by *Mycobacterium ulcerans*.
(d) History and appearance are characteristic. Isolation of the organism may be achieved in embryonated hens' eggs; serological tests are not very helpful.
(e) It will heal within 2–3 weeks.

152 (a) It consists of pustules distributed over the lateral aspect of the pinna. The appearance is consistent with herpes simplex. A similar rash may be found in herpes zoster involving the geniculate ganglion of the seventh

cranial nerve but the distribution is more restricted to the skin around the external auditory meatus.
(b) *Herpesvirus hominis* type I.
(c) A recurent attack of herpes simplex infection is often precipitated by intercurrent infection and is particularly common in septic meningitis, certain forms of pneumonia and malaria.
(d) Testing for circulating antibody is valuable in primary infection but is unhelpful in recurrent infections because pre-existing antibody titre may not change.

153 (a) He has cellulitis.
(b) Fever, rigor, pain and swelling of the groin.
(c) Erysipelas, primary or secondary to lymphatic obstruction; perhaps caused by Bancroftian filariasis.
(d) Yes, lymphoedema with tendency to further attacks of cellulitis, which may or may not be infective in origin; elephatiasis.

154 (a) Risus sardonicus.
(b) Tetanus.
(c) The spores of *Clostridium tetani* gain entry through a wound, existing abrasion or ulcer, or placental bed.
(d) The shorter the incubation period, the higher the case fatality. The shorter the period of onset, which is the time from the first symptom to the first spasm, the higher the case fatality.
(e) Yes. Nursing care, sedation and specific treatment can alter the mortality, which in many series has exceeded 50 per cent.

155 (a) A large mediastinal mass showing calcification at its edge. This is an aortic aneurysm involving the ascending part, the arch and the descending thoracic aorta. There is marked cardiac enlargement.
(b) A diastolic murmur at the base of the heart.
(c) Syphilitic. Treponemal serology was strongly positive.
(d) *Treponema pallidum* affects the small vessels of the wall of the aorta, with destruction of elastic tissue and deposition of fibrous tissue. The aorta dilates and this involves the aortic ring, giving rise to aortic incompetence with strain on the left ventricle, as suggested by the cardiac enlargement. The dilated aorta compresses the left recurrent laryngeal nerve, causing hoarseness, while compression of the trachea results in coughing.
(e) Poor. Once left ventricular failure develops it tends to be intractable. Death may be due to rupture of the aneurysm.

156 (a) Measles.
(b) No. It is unusual for a drug-induced rash to evolve in this manner.
(c) Congestion of the conjunctivae and buccal mucosa; generalised enlargement of lymph nodes.
(d) Otitis media, pneumonia or encephalitis.

157 (a) Polymorphonuclear leucocytes and Gram-negative diplococci—*Neisseria meningitidis*.
(b) More than 1000 polymorphonuclear leucocytes/mm^3.
(c) The CSF protein is likely to be 1g/l or more and the CSF sugar less than half the blood sugar level.
(d) The organism can be cultured from the blood in approximately half the patients with meningococcal meningitis.
(e) Yes, in approximately half the patients.

158 (a) Hepatic carcinoma, cirrhosis and amoebic liver abscess, although the latter is unlikely in view of the duration of symptoms and lack of liver tenderness.
(b) Liver biopsy will establish the diagnosis but should be carried out with care since bleeding may occur.
(c) In the developing world, hepatitis B virus infection is associated strongly with hepatoma and there is evidence for a causative relationship.
(d) In areas where hepatitis B virus infection is common, transmission is often from mother to infant at delivery. Vaccination of the infants of hepatitis-B-positive mothers may offer some protection. Improvement in general standards of hygiene may be expected to result in a reduction in this infection.
(e) Very poor. Major surgical procedures and cytotoxic drugs would have little benefit. The appearance of jaundice is a terminal event.

159 (a) A fungus, *Madurella mycetomi*, is the cause of Madura foot.
(b) It is thought that fungi in the soil enter through an abrasion in the skin.
(c) The appearance is characteristic, especially if grains, which in this case were black, are seen in the discharge.
(d) The infection may spread locally up the leg or to deeper tissues. Distal spread does not usually occur.
(e) An X-ray of the foot may be entirely normal. If bone is involved, the appearance is confused with that of chronic bacterial osteomyelitis.

160 (a) Calcification of the bladder.
(b) The calcification is of schistosome ova in the wall of the bladder.
(c) Nil. The appearances are pathognomonic of urinary schistosomiasis.
(d) Local: papilloma and carcinoma of the bladder; hydronephrosis with reduced renal function. Distal: ova carried embolically to the lungs may give rise to pulmonary hypertension.

161 (a) A varicella vesicle is present on the conjunctiva. Lesions can be seen on the adjacent skin.
(b) A conjunctival lesion from the varicella usually resolves spontaneously with no residual damage.

162 (a) Yes. An eschar from a tick bite is commonly present and is usually associated with regional lymphadenitis.
(b) Tick typhus.
(c) *Rickettsia conori*.
(d) Rarely.
(e) Tick typhus of the Old World is a benign illness with a low mortality.

163 (a) Herpes zoster and a generalised rash of varicella, the appearance of which has been modified by scratching.
(b) She also has jaundice, a distended abdomen with an umbilical hernia and has had bilateral mastectomies.
(c) Carcinoma of the breast with metastases. This has resulted in impaired immunity and reactivation of latent *Herpesvirus varicellae/zoster*.

164 (a) The symptoms and the presence of a vesicular rash in the posterior half of the mouth point to herpangina.
(b) Viruses of Coxsackie group A.
(c) The fever settles after 4 days; the vesicles rupture and leave shallow ulcers, which heal within 1 week.

165 (a) A microfilaria of *Onchocerca volvolus*; the tip of the tail is free of nuclei and the parasite has no sheath.
(b) Because the infection often involves the eye, giving rise to a punctuate keratitis which may become irreversible and lead to blindness.

(c) Treatment, which damages microfilariae, is followed by an increase in skin lesions and eye symptoms.

(d) Yes, if the adult worms are killed by treatment. If only microfilariae are damaged, symptoms may return after some weeks or months.

(e) Transmission from man to man is by Simulium (black) flies. Control consists of reduction in man–fly contact and measures against the fly, which breeds in water.

166 (a) Branching filaments of *Actinomyces*.

(b) *Actinomyces* are Gram-positive bacteria. They are not fungi and reproduce by division and not by the formation of spores or budding.

(c) The 'sulphur granule', formed by a mass of mycelia held together by calcium phosphate.

(d) Probably through the neglected teeth.

(e) Good, apart from the effect of fibrosis. The organism is sensitive to many antibiotics, which need to be given for weeks to reach bacteria within fibrotic tissue and granules. Chemotherapy should be used, together with surgery to drain abscesses or excise sinuses.

167 (a) The symptoms are consistent with either Stevens–Johnson syndrome or toxic epidermal necrolysis (scalded-skin syndrome). The absence of pain in the skin points to the former.

(b) A hypersensitivity response to infection or drugs.

(c) The acute phase usually lasts 7–10 days then the lesions gradually resolve. A complete recovery is usual.

(d) Joints, lungs, myo- and pericardium, brain and small bowel.

168 (a) Dengue haemorrhagic fever.

(b) A dengue virus, belonging to the *Togavirus* family and the *Flavivirus* genus. There are four serotypes.

(c) By mosquito bite. *Aedes aegypti* is the most important vector; it breeds readily in small collections of relatively clean water lying in containers around homes.

(d) Hypovolaemic shock is a serious and common complication in children with repeated dengue infection who live in South East Asia.

169 (a) Vincent's angina.

(b) A spirochaete, *Borrelia vincentii*, and a fusiform bacillus, *Fusobacterium fusiforme*. They are easily detected in smears but are difficult to culture.

(c) They do not usually act as primary pathogens but as secondary invaders when superficial tissues have been damaged or are defective as a result of trauma, other infection, malnutrition, agranulocytosis or leukaemia.

170 (a) Probably *Neisseria meningitidis*.

(b) Arthritis which usually develops at a late stage and involves large joints.

(c) Fluid aspirated is viscous and contains pus cells but organisms are seldom found.

(d) Usually, uneventful with no residual disability.

171 (a) Desquamation—shedding of the surface layers of the stratum corneum.

(b) No. It may be found after any intensely erythematous rash.

(c) Usually on the trunk.

(d) No.

172 (a) The chest X-ray shows a mediastinal mass—probably enlarged mediastinal lymph nodes. They may be caused by tuberculosis, lymphoma or sarcoidosis; less probably by aortic aneurysm, tumour or congenital cyst.
(b) If caused by tuberculosis, the tuberculin test would be strongly positive and may even ulcerate; if caused by sarcoidosis, the Kveim test would be positive.
(c) Only if caused by tuberculosis; usually acid-fast bacilli are not seen.
(d) It might indicate lymphoma. In disseminated tuberculosis acid-fast organisms may be found but this is unlikely in tuberculous mediastinal glands.
(e) Mediastinoscopy with biopsy may provide histological and often bacteriological confirmation of tuberculous glands. In this young Asian the most probable diagnosis is tuberculosis.

173 (a) Oocysts of cryptosporidium.
(b) Auramine, Giemsa or a modified Ziehl–Neelsen, which has been used here.
(c) Domestic animals, including dogs and cats, meat or meat products, and infected individuals, especially children.

174 (a) Osteomyelitis involving C6 and 7 with loss of intervertebral space. A marked feature is the new bone formation on the anterior surface of C6, which almost forms a bridge to C7. This is called 'beaking'.
(b) Tuberculosis and brucellosis. Beaking is a feature of brucellosis.
(c) No, the lesions are usually single.
(d) No, the lesions are permanent.
(e) Although serological tests would suggest the cause, a firm diagnosis would require a biopsy.

175 (a) It is erythema marginatum and is a hypersensitivity response to infection with *Streptococcus pyogenes*.
(b) Rheumatic fever.
(c) There is no specific test for rheumatic fever but the erythrocyte sedimentation test is markedly raised and the anti-streptolysin O titre is high.
(d) Rheumatic fever as such is not infectious but the patient may still be harbouring *Streptococcus pyogenes* in his nose or throat and may spread this infection to others.

176 (a) The prodromal period of pain and the unilateral distribution of the eruption points to a diagnosis of herpes zoster, involving the second division of the fifth cranial nerve.
(b) Yes, on the left side of his face over the maxilla.
(c) The blisters on the palate will rupture to leave shallow ulceration which will heal without scab formation.
(d) Many patients will have troublesome post-herpetic neuralgia.

177 (a) A schizont of *Plasmodium malariae*, showing division of the parent parasite into about eight developing merozoites; this is characteristic of this species of malarial parasite.
(b) It is impossible to know. *P. malariae*, infection may be very long-lived; initial infection may have been at any time in the tropics.
(c) Fever and headaches are common to all malaria infections; the periodicity of *P. malariae* is 72 hours. His splenomegaly and mild anaemia may both be caused by the malaria infection.
(d) It will end the current attack and would be expected to eradicate the infection. It is thought that *P. malariae* does not have persisting liver forms (exoerythrocytic forms) and that 'relapses' are really recrudescences due to persisting blood forms.

(e) *P. malariae* infections have been associated with nephropathy giving rise to nephrotic syndrome in children; also associated with tropical splenomegaly syndrome, although the spleen is often much larger than in this patient.

178 (a) This may be caused by herpes simplex infection or by infection with Vincent's organisms. In herpetic gingivitis discrete vesicles form on the gums but soon run together and burst to form serpiginous ulcers. Herpetic lesions may be found on the lips and elsewhere. In Vincent's infection there is destruction of the interdental papillae, resulting shallow concave ulcers with white necrotic margins.
(b) Yes.
(c) Clinical assessment is usually sufficient. Laboratory confirmation may be obtained by culturing the virus or by demonstrating a rise in antibody level.
(d) He is unlikely to have further episodes of herpetic gingivitis. However, one in three patients will suffer from recurrent attacks involving the lips at the mucocutaneous junction.

179 (a) Congenital rubella.
(b) Deafness and cataract. These defects in conjunction with congenital heart disease constitute the rubella triad.
(c) Rubella virus may be recovered readily from throat secretions and cerebrospinal fluid at birth and may be found also in urine, faeces and blood. Up to 20 per cent of children with congential rubella may still be shedding virus at 15 months and 5 per cent at 18 months.

180 (a) Tuberculosis lymphadenitis. Tuberculosis of the cervical lymph nodes is also known as scrofula.
(b) It has been reported in 5–12 per cent of patients.
(c) *Mycobacterium tuberculosis* or *bovis* depending upon the environment. In the USA *M. tuberculosis* is more commonly found.
(d) The accessory nerve has been damaged, with resulting wasting of the trapezius on the right.

181 (a) A parasite cut across transversely and lying in a bile duct.
(b) Yes. Biliary obstruction by the trematode *Clonorchis sinensis* predisposes to cholangitis. In this patient *E. coli* was responsible, while in others a salmonella may be grown from the blood.
(c) Eggs passed into water are ingested by snails, in which they hatch into miracidia. Large numbers of cercariae are later released, which penetrate beneath the scales of certain fish. If the fish are eaten raw or undercooked man becomes infected. The parasite passes up the bile duct.
(d) No. The majority of those infected with *C. sinensis* are asymptomatic.
(e) In those with clonorchiasis there is an increased incidence of cholangio-carcinoma.

182 (a) A long stricture of the transverse colon.
(b) Crohn's disease. There is a suggestion of some fissuring.
(c) Tissue diagnosis is essential.
(d) Granulomatous inflammation. This proved to be caused by tuberculosis.

183 (a) Thrush, or oral candidiasis.
(b) A yeast, *Candida albicans*.
(c) In adults infection is usually endogenous; in infants it may result from cross-infection.
(d) They include dehydration, debility, chemotherapy and immunodeficiency.

184 (a) Scabies.

(b) It is particularly prominent around interdigital spaces, on backs of hands, wrists, axillae, groins, breasts, umbilicus, penis and buttocks.

(c) A mite, *Sarcoptes scabei*.

(d) Human; animal mites do not establish themselves in man.

(e) Usually by direct contact but also by bedding and clothing if infestation is severe; sexual contact.

185 (a) The site of the lesion, the slow progression over many years and the onset in childhood suggest lupus vulgaris. Other chronic granulomata of the skin include leprosy, leishmaniasis and mycoses.

(b) By skin biopsy. Tubercles may be demonstrated in the dermis, but tubercle bacilli, although present, are rarely seen and can be cultured in only 50 per cent of cases.

(c) By direct inoculation of the skin with tubercle bacilli. A case of active pulmonary tuberculosis may be found in the household.

(d) Untreated lupus persists indefinitely. It spreads centrifugally but very slowly and is never the direct cause of death. Pulmonary tuberculosis may occur as a terminal event.

186 (a) Acute ulcerative gingivitis.

(b) Vincent's organisms—a spirochaete, *Borrelia vincentii*, and fusiform bacillus, *Fusobacterium fusiforme*.

(c) Vincent's organisms act as secondary invaders; when superficial tissues have been damaged or are defective as a result of trauma, other infections, malnutrition, agranulocytosis or leukaemia.

187 (a) A gumma. A gummatous ulcer is characteristically painless and has well-defined 'punched-out' edges. The base is indurated and is covered by a firmly adherent slough of necrotic tissue, resembling a piece of wash-leather.

(b) Spirochaetes are difficult to detect in the lesion. Syphilis serology would be positive and there would be a rapid therapeutic response to penicillin.

(c) Gummata are a late manifestation of syphilis and may appear as early as 1 year after the primary infection but are more likely to develop after an interval of several years. Eventually a gumma will heal spontaneously, leaving a paper-thin atrophic non-contractile scar.

(d) A gumma is a granulomatous lesion with a marked degree of obliterative endarteritis involving the small vessels. There is infiltration of endothelial cells and lymphocytes with giant cells similar to those found in tuberculosis surrounded by a zone of fibrous tissue.

188 (a) No. The swelling is too low and too far back for the parotid gland.

(b) A suppurative lymphadenitis. This is not infrequently mistaken for mumps in a young child.

(c) Many cases are due to infection with *Staphylococcus aureus* and there is seldom any obvious portal of entry; some are caused by *Streptococcus pyogenes* and are secondary to tonsillitis.

(d) A polymorphonuclear leucocytosis.

189 (a) The chest X-ray shows opacities with a ground-glass appearance fanning out from the hilum. This appearance may be found in mycoplasmal infection, ornithosis, Q fever and a number of virus infections, including respiratory syncytial virus, adenovirus, parainfluenza virus and influenza virus. However, the slow onset of the illness, the disparity between the X-ray appearance and the physical signs, the high ESR and the presence of cold agglutinins favour a diagnosis of mycoplasmal pneumonia.

(b) *Mycoplasma pneumoniae*, a cell-wall-deficient organism.

(c) Fever gradually subsides after 7–10 days. Convalescence is slow, and radiological changes may persist for weeks.

(d) By demonstrating a fourfold rise in antibodies against mycoplasma.

(e) Haemolytic anaemia, arthritis, myocarditis, encephalitis, myelitis and polyneuritis.

190 (a) Kaposi's sarcoma. The European variety of the disease has a peak incidence in the sixth and seventh decades, whereas the African variety reaches a peak in the third decade and has a much higher incidence of visceral involvement.

(b) Generalised lymphadenopathy and the early emergence of Kaposi's sarcoma point to acquired immune deficiency syndrome.

(c) Skin biopsy to confirm the diagnosis and antibody test for HIV infection. A chest X-ray may show pneumonitis.

(d) Hopeless when associated with AIDS.

191 (a) A coiled larva.

(b) This is the larva of *Trichinella spiralis*. The diarrhoea was related to the development of adult worms in the gut, The general symptoms. periorbital oedema and eosinophilia are related to migration of larvae from the gut lumen through tissues. The myalgia is related to encystment of larvae in muscles.

(c) By eating undercooked meat, most commonly pork. The cyst wall is digested in the stomach and the larva matures to an adult in the gut lumen.

(d) Serum antibodies are detectable but usually not before the third week.

(e) Good. Most infections are asymptomatic. When there is illness the symptoms subside after a few weeks. Occasionally a patient may die from myocarditis.

192 (a) Aseptic meningitis. The history of contact with a young dog and the conjunctival suffusion point to leptospirosis rather than a virus infection.

(b) *Leptospira canicola*. Humans may be infected from dogs, pigs and other animals.

(c) The leptospires may be found in the CSF during the first week of illness but disappear rapidly as antibodies form.

(d) Serologically, by a fourfold rise in antibodies.

(e) No. Renal failure seldom occurs in man although it is a feature of the infection in the dog.

193 (a) Developing trophozoite of *Plasmodium malariae*.

(b) There is a strong association between the nephrotic syndrome in children and *P. malariae* infection.

(c) Immune-complex deposition on the glomerular basement membrane, resulting in heavy proteinuria, greatly reduced serum albumin and oedema.

(d) A schizontocide will eradicate malaria infection but will have little effect on the renal lesion.

(e) Poor. Treatment is less effective than in the nephrotic syndrome of temperate climates.

194 (a) An enanthen consisting of petechiae on the palate and an exudative tonsillitis.

(b) Infectious mononucleosis. It would be unusual to have this degree of fever in diphtheria and diphtheritic membrane may extend off the tonsils to the palate. A petechial enanthem of this type is most unusual in diphtheria.

(c) Generalised enlargement of lymph nodes, splenomegaly and possibly mild jaundice.

(d) By finding atypical mononuclear cells in the peripheral blood and by demonstrating heterophil antibodies to sheep or horse red blood cells.

195 (a) She has suffered an aplastic crisis.

(b) Patients with homozygous sickle-cell disease have a low haemoglobin level but a high reticulocyte count. The present low reticulocyte count indicates lack of delivery of red blood cells to the peripheral circulation. Since circulating red blood cells have such a short lifespan, a sudden fall in haemoglobin results.

(c) Infection or red cell precursors with parvovirus.

(d) Yes, painful crises, often precipitated by infection generally, but she is unlikely to have a further aplastic crisis because parvovirus infection gives rise to immunity.

(e) This is one of the few circumstances in which a patient with sickle-cell disease should be transfused.

196 (a) Erythema infectiosum (Fifth disease). The cheeks appear to have been slapped, hence the other synonym of slapped-cheek syndrome. The rash on the limbs has a lace-like appearance with a tendency to come-and-go.

(b) Infection with a parvovirus.

(c) Yes and tends to be more severe. It may be accompanied by arthritis and enlargement of lymph nodes.

(d) The illness follows a benign course and complications are rare.

197 (a) This rests between disseminated gonococcal infection and chronic meningococcal septicaemia. A pustular rash is more frequently found in the former but haemorrhagic, macular or papular lesions may be found in both. This is gonococcal.

(b) The organism may be grown from blood or from synovial fluid in about 50 per cent of cases. Blood culture is most rewarding during the first week and synovial fluid culture once the arthritis has become frankly purulent.

(c) It may be genital, rectal or pharyngeal.

(d) It is asymptomatic in 80 per cent of cases in both men and women.

(e) Tenosynovitis is found in about 25 per cent of cases and endocarditis is about 3 per cent.

198 (a) Nodal bradycardia with ventricular ectopic escape, depression of the S–T segment and inversion of T waves.

(b) Diphtheria of the throat.

(c) Diphtheria toxin damages both the myocardium and the motor nerves. Evidence of heart damage appears first, followed by palatal and other palsies begining about days 14–21.

(d) When heart damage is severe, death commonly occurs about the 15th day. If the patient survives, ultimate recovery is assured.

199 (a) The possibility of cat-scratch disease should always be considered in a patient with unexplained lymphadenitis when there is a history of exposure to cats. In cat-scratch disease the epitrochlear, axillary and cervical groups are most frequently involved. Lymphangitis is not a feature and the primary lesion at the site of injury may be absent. Other causes of lymphadenitis would be unlikely to affect such an unusual distribution of nodes.

(b) By a specific skin test using an antigen prepared from sterilised diluted bubo pus.

(c) Ultimate recovery but the course of the illness is variable and may be prolonged. It is never fatal.

200 (a) Ova of *Ascaris lumbricoides,* the human roundworm.

(b) None. Roundworms do not produce symptoms of this kind.

(c) Yes. Tests of absorption would be appropriate.

(d) *Giardia lamblia* infection may produce malabsorption and the trophozoites may be found on jejunal aspirate even when the parasite is not demonstrated in the stool.

(e) Tropical sprue with an ascaris infection.

INDEX

Numbers refer to illustrations